# Shoulder Rehabilitation

## Non-Operative Treatment

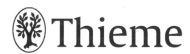

# Shoulder Rehabilitation

## Non-Operative Treatment

Todd S. Ellenbecker, D.P.T., M.S., S.C.S., O.C.S., C.S.C.S.
Clinic Director
Physiotherapy Associates Scottsdale Sports Clinic
Scottsdale, Arizona
National Director of Clinical Research
Physiotherapy Associates
Memphis, Tennessee

Thieme
New York • Stuttgart

# Dedication

To Gail for her constant support and love.

Thieme Medical Publishers, Inc.
333 Seventh Ave.
New York, NY 10001

Associate Editor: Birgitta Brandenburg
Vice President, Production and Electronic Publishing: Anne T. Vinnicombe
Production Editor: Print Matters, Inc.
Sales Director: Ross Lumpkin
Associate Marketing Director: Verena Diem
Chief Financial Officer: Peter van Woerden
President: Brian D. Scanlan
Compositor: Alden Books

Printer: CPI books, Leck
Cover photograph: Lance Jeffrey/US Tennis Association
Library of Congress Cataloging-in-Publication Data

Shoulder rehabilitation : non-operative treatment / [edited by] Todd
S. Ellenbecker.
    p. : cm.
    Includes bibliographical references and index.
    ISBN 1-58890-370-2 (US/HC) — ISBN 3-13-140221-0 (GTV/HC)
    1. Shoulder—Wounds and injuries—Treatment. 2. Shoulder—Pathophysiology. I.
Ellenbecker, Todd S., 1962.
    [DNLM: 1. Shoulder—injuries. 2. Rehabilitation—methods. 3.
Shoulder—physiopathology, 4. Shoulder Joint—injuries. 5. Shoulder
Joint—physiopathology. WE 810 S55868 2006]
    RD557.5.S56 2006
    617.5'72044—dc22

                                                                2006043874

**Important note:** Medical knowledge is ever-changing. As new research and clinical experience broaden our knowledge, changes in treatment and drug therapy may be required. The authors and editors of the material herein have consulted sources believed to be reliable in their efforts to provide information that is complete and in accord with the standards accepted at the time of publication. However, in view of the possibility of human error by the authors, editors, or publisher of the work herein or changes in medical knowledge, neither the authors, editors, or publisher, nor any other party who has been involved in the preparation of this work, warrants that the information contained herein is in every respect accurate or complete, and they are not responsible for any errors or omissions or for the results obtained from use of such information. Readers are encouraged to confirm the information contained herein with other sources. For example, readers are advised to check the product information sheet included in the package of each drug they plan to administer to be certain that the information contained in this publication is accurate and that changes have not been made in the recommended dose or in the contraindications for administration. This recommendation is of particular importance in connection with new or infrequently used drugs.

Some of the product names, patents, and registered designs referred to in this book are in fact registered trademarks or proprietary names even though specific reference to this fact is not always made in the text. Therefore, the appearance of a name without designation as proprietary is not to be construed as a representation by the publisher that it is in the public domain.

Printed in Germany

5 4 3 2 1

TMP ISBN 1-58890-370-2
        978-1-58890-370-9
GTV ISBN 3 13 140221 0
        978-3-13-140221-9

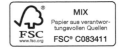

# Contents

# Foreword

As a person who has been involved with both the basic science and clinical application of shoulder rehabilitation for many years, I know how diverse and challenging a topic this is. The shoulder is a tough joint to study, and it is difficult to completely rehabilitate due to the high forces and loads, large motions, and repetitive nature of its use.

To that end, many books have been written to discuss and present rehabilitation protocols. What makes this book different is its approach: emphasizing the importance of rehabilitation as a means of restoring optimal function to the shoulder. This restoration requires several elements, which are outlined and developed in the book. First is the grounding of the exercises and protocols in basic science and clinical research so that there is evidence for the efficacy of the exercises and protocols. Second, the restoration is accomplished by emphasis on kinetic chain evaluation and kinetic chain-based protocols. Efficient kinetic chain activation is the basis for optimal shoulder function and should be the end goal for all the rehabilitation exercises.

Third, this book emphasizes "let the body guide you"—marking progress and instituting progressions on the basis of demonstrated functional capabilities in the kinetic chain, rather than a specific timetable. In this way, the body is ready for each new exercise challenge. Finally, it is not a one-size-fits-all book. Sport-specific protocols are outlined to allow adjustment of the final stages in the rehabilitation sequence in order to ensure that the patient is ready for the unique demands of the particular sport or activity. This book will be of great value to doctors and therapists in their efforts to restore optimal shoulder function. Todd Ellenbecker has assembled a distinguished group of researchers and clinicians, and the reader will benefit from their expertise in this area.

*W. Ben Kibler, M.D.*
*Medical Director*
*Lexington Clinic Sports Medicine Center*
*Lexington, Kentucky*

# Preface

Rehabilitating the patient with an injured shoulder requires an exhaustive knowledge of basic science and clinical evidence. The purpose of this book is to integrate this information for the most common shoulder diagnoses in a format that combines the latest evidence with helpful photographs and technical guidance from experts in the field.

The first section of this book covers the most common diagnoses seen in orthopaedic and sports physical therapy clinics for which nonoperative rehabilitation is provided. Each chapter integrates basic science and clinical research to advance the understanding of the structures being treated. The complex biomechanics of the human shoulder are coupled with the latest evidence-based rehabilitation strategies. Unlike texts that contain protocols for postoperative rehabilitation, this book features progressions and principles for treatment that take into account the often varied rates of recovery and severities of injury seen in patients presenting for nonoperative treatment.

Ben Kibler's chapter in the first section outlines the challenges in evaluating and treating the scapulothoracic joint for virtually all types of shoulder patients. His keen insight and cutting-edge evaluation and classification techniques, combined with evidence-based exercise progressions, can be applied to each of the chapters outlining specific treatment for shoulder pathology. This kinetic chain approach to rehabilitation is a recurring theme in virtually all of the chapters and represents the advancement of the "whole extremity" or "total arm strength" treatment philosophy that has developed over the past decade to an advanced understanding and interpretation of biomechanical research and the kinetic chain. It can no longer be thought acceptable to simply strengthen an isolated segment of the body during rehabilitation without considering the adjoining segments and ultimately the entire body through its kinetic chain during rehabilitation.

The final section of the text provides greater detail on a series of important topics encountered during rehabilitation of the patient with an injured shoulder, namely, the return to full activity. These chapters include detailed treatment of such topics as the return to safe and productive weightlifting through a program with anatomically and biomechanically based modifications, as well as the use of taping and bracing. The final chapter deals with interval return to sport guidelines and contains sport- and activity-specific details in addition to actual programs drafted by therapists who work with athletes at all levels within those specific sports. The most common shoulder-related sports are included in this helpful chapter.

# Acknowledgments

We thank the authors of this book for their dedication to their field, and for agreeing to share the latest science and evidence and their clinical mastery in the development of these chapters. Thanks to Thieme Medical Publishing and Birgitta Brandenburg and her staff for giving us this incredible opportunity to put this information on shoulder rehabilitation together. Finally, we are grateful to our shoulder patients and mentors without whom we would never have gained the knowledge and insight to be able to complete this project.

# Contributors

James R. Andrews, M.D.
Orthopedic Surgeon
Alabama Sports Medicine & Orthopedic Center
Chairman and Medical Director
American Sports Medicine Institute
Birmingham, Alabama

Jake Bleacher, M.S., P.T., O.C.S., C.S.C.S.
Physiotherapy Associates Gilbert Sports Clinic
Gilbert, Arizona

George J. Davies, P.T., D.P.T., S.C.S., M.Ed.
  A.T.C., C.S.C.S.
Armstrong Atlantic University
Physical Therapy Department,
Savannah, Georgia

Christine E. Di Lorenzo, P.T.
Director
West Side Physical Therapy
New York, New York

Todd S. Ellenbecker, D.P.T., M.S., S.C.S.,
  O.C.S., C.S.C.S.
Clinic Director
Physiotherapy Associates Scottsdale Sports Clinic
Scottsdale, Arizona
National Director of Clinical Research
Physiotherapy Associates
Memphis, Tennessee

Charles Hazle, M.S., P.T.
Assistant Professor
University of Kentucky
Center for Rural Health
Hazard, Kentucky

Jason Jennings, D.P.T., S.C.S., A.T.C., M.T.C., C.S.C.S.
Medical Student
Tampa, Florida

W. Ben Kibler, M.D.
Medical Director
Lexington Clinic Sports Medicine Center
Lexington, Kentucky

Leonard C. Macrina, M.S.P.T., C.S.C.S.
Physical Therapist
Champion Sports Medicine
Birmingham, Alabama

Terry R. Malone, Ed.D., P.T., A.T.C.
Director of Physical therapy
University of Kentucky
Lexington, Kentucky

Rob Manske, D.P.T., M.Ed., S.C.S., A.T.C., C.S.C.S.
Assistant Professor
Wichita State University
Wichita, Kansas

James W. Matheson, D.P.T., M.S., P.T.,
  S.C.S., C.S.C.S.
Clinical Research Director
Therapy Partners, Inc.
Maplewood, Minnesota

Michael J. Mullaney, M.P.T.
Senior Physical Therapist/Research Assistant
NISMAT at Lenox Hill Hospital
New York, New York

Timothy F. Murphy, P.T.
President
Concorde Therapy Group
Canton, Ohio

Russ Morgan Paine, P.T.
Director
Sports Rehab Centers of Houston
Benchmark Medical
Rehabilitation Consultant
Houston Astros, Houston Rockets, NASA
Houston, Texas

Michael M. Reinold, P.T., D.P.T., A.T.C., C.S.C.S.
Assistant Athletic Trainer
Boston Red Sox Baseball Club
Adjunct Faculty
Northeastern University
Boston, Massachusetts

Robert Schulte, D.H.Sc., P.T., S.C.S.
Associate Professor
University of Mary
Bismark, North Dakota

Anna E. Thatcher, M.S., P.T., A.T.C.
Physical Therapist
Physiotherapy Associates Scottsdale Sports Clinic
Scottsdale, Arizona

Timothy F. Tyler, P.T., A.T.C.
Clinical Research Associate
NISMAT at Lenox Hill Hospital
New York, New York
PRO Sports Physical Therapy of Westchester
Scarsdale, New York

Kevin E. Wilk, P.T.
Vice President of Education—Benchmark
    Medical
Clinic Director
Champion Sports Medicine
Birmingham, Alabama
Adjunct Faculty
Marquette University
Milwaukee, Wisconsin

# I

# Rehabilitation of Specific Shoulder Pathologies

# 1

# Rehabilitation of Shoulder Impingement: Primary, Secondary, and Internal

**Todd S. Ellenbecker**

To rehabilitate the patient with glenohumeral joint impingement requires a careful, systematic evaluation to identify the type of impingement and, more importantly, to determine the underlying cause of the impingement to ensure that an evidence-based nonoperative rehabilitation program can be developed. Significant advances in basic research in the anatomy and biomechanics of the human shoulder have led to the identification of multiple types of impingement, each with underlying pathomechanical causes. In this chapter, the main types of rotator cuff impingement are discussed together with both general and specific rehabilitation principles and strategies based on the available evidence.

## ◆ Types of Rotator Cuff Impingement

### Primary Impingement or Compressive Disease

Primary impingement, also known as *compressive disease* or *outlet impingement,* is a direct result of compression of the rotator cuff tendons between the humeral head and the overlying anterior third of the acromion, coracoacromial ligament, coracoid, or acromial-clavicular joint.[1,2] The physiologic space between the inferior acromion and superior surface of the rotator cuff tendons is termed the subacromial space. Measured using anteroposterior radiographs, it was 7 to 13 mm in size in patients with shoulder pain[3] and 6 to 14 mm in normal shoulders.[4] Flatow et al[5] have shown that elevation of the humerus leads to predictable and reproducible patterns of subacromial impingement of the rotator cuff tendons against the overlying acromion and coracoacromial ligament.

Biomechanical analysis of the shoulder has produced theoretical estimates of the compressive forces against the acromion with elevation of the shoulder. Poppen and Walker[6] calculated this force at 0.42 times body weight. Lucas[7] estimated this force at 10.2 times the weight of the arm. Peak forces against the acromion were measured in a range of motion (ROM) between 85 degrees and 136 degrees of elevation.[8] This position is a functionally important one for daily activities, sport-specific movements,[9,10] and situations commonly encountered on a job as well. The position of the shoulder in forward flexion, horizontal adduction, and internal rotation (IR) during the acceleration and follow-through phases of the throwing motion is likely to produce subacromial impingement due to abrasion of the supraspinatus, infraspinatus, or biceps tendon against the overlying structures.[9] These data provide scientific rationale for the concept of primary impingement or compressive disease as an etiology of rotator cuff pathology.

### Neer's Stages of Impingement

Neer[1,2] has outlined three stages of primary impingement as it relates to rotator cuff pathology.

*Stage I—edema and hemorrhage—*results from the mechanical irritation of the tendon; this is caused by impingement incurred from overhead activity. Observed in younger, more athletic patients, it is a reversible condition with conservative physical therapy. The primary symptoms and physical signs of this stage of impingement or compressive disease are similar to the other two stages and consist of a positive impingement sign, painful arc of movement, and varying degrees of muscular weakness.[2]

*Stage II compressive disease* outlined by Neer is termed *fibrosis and tendonitis.* This occurs from repeated episodes of mechanical inflammation and can include thickening or fibrosis of the subacromial bursae. The typical age range for this stage of injury is 25 to 40 years.

Neer's *stage III impingement lesion,* termed *bone spurs and tendon rupture,* is the result of continued mechanical compression of the rotator cuff tendons. Full-thickness tears of the rotator cuff, partial-thickness tears of the rotator cuff, biceps tendon lesions, and bony alteration of the acromion and acromioclavicular joint may be associated with this stage.[1,2] In addition to bony alterations that are acquired with repetitive stress to the shoulder, the native shape of the acromion is of relevance.

The specific shape of the overlying acromion process is termed *acromial architecture* and has been studied in relation to full-thickness tears of the rotator cuff.[11,12] Bigliani et al[11] described three types of acromions: type I (flat), type II (curved), and type III (hooked). A type III or hooked acromion was found in 70% of cadaveric shoulders with a full-thickness rotator cuff tear, whereas a type I acromion was only associated with 3% of this group.[11] Additionally, in a series of 200 clinically evaluated patients, 80% with a positive arthrogram confirming a full-thickness rotator cuff tear had a type III acromion.[12]

## Secondary Impingement

Impingement or compressive symptoms may be secondary to underlying instability of the glenohumeral joint.[13,14] Though relatively common knowledge today, this concept was not well understood or recognized in the medical community even through the mid- to late 1980s. The development of the concept that impingement could occur secondary to instability, rather than as a primary cause, has had significant ramifications altering evaluation methods and treatment/rehabilitation.[15,16]

Attenuation of the static stabilizers of the glenohumeral joint, such as the capsular ligaments and labrum from the excessive demands incurred in throwing or overhead activities, can lead to anterior instability of the glenohumeral joint. Due to the increased humeral head translation, the biceps tendon and rotator cuff can become impinged secondary to the ensuing instability.[13,14] A progressive loss of glenohumeral joint stability is created when the dynamic stabilizing functions of the rotator cuff are diminished from fatigue and tendon injury.[14,17] The effects of secondary impingement can lead to rotator cuff tears as the instability and impingement continue.[3,14]

## Posterior, Internal, or Undersurface Impingement

An additional type of impingement more recently discussed as an etiology for rotator cuff pathology that can often progress to an undersurface tear of the rotator cuff in the shoulder of a young athletic patient is termed *posterior, internal or inside, or undersurface* impingement.[18,19] This phenomenon was originally identified by Walch et al[19] upon performing shoulder arthroscopy with the shoulder placed in the 90 degrees of abduction

and 90 degrees of external rotation (ER) (90/90) position. Placement of the shoulder in the 90/90 position causes the supraspinatus and infraspinatus tendons to rotate posteriorly. This more-posterior orientation of the tendons aligns them such that the undersurface of the tendons rubs on the posterior-superior glenoid lip and becomes pinched or compressed between the humeral head and the posterosuperior glenoid rim.[19] In contrast to patients with traditional outlet impingement (either primary or secondary), the area of the rotator cuff tendon that is involved in posterior or undersurface impingement is the articular side of the rotator cuff tendon. Traditional impingement involves the superior or bursal surface of the rotator cuff tendon or tendons and typically produces anterior and anterolateral pain distributions.[20] Conversely, individuals presenting with posterior shoulder pain brought on by positioning of the arm in 90 degrees of abduction and 90 degrees or more of ER, typically from overhead positions in sport or work activities, may be considered as potential candidates for undersurface impingement.

The presence of anterior translation of the humeral head with maximal ER and 90 degrees of abduction, which has been confirmed arthroscopically during the subluxation-relocation test, can produce mechanical rubbing and fraying on the undersurface of the rotator cuff tendons. There can be additional harm caused by the posterior deltoid if the rotator cuff is not functioning properly. The posterior deltoid's angle of pull compresses the humeral head against the glenoid, accentuating the skeletal, tendinous, and labral lesions.[18] Walch et al[19] arthroscopically evaluated 17 throwing athletes with shoulder pain during throwing and found undersurface impingement that resulted in eight partial-thickness rotator cuff tears and 12 lesions in the posterosuperior labrum. Impingement of the undersurface of the rotator cuff on the posterosuperior glenoid labrum may be a cause of painful structural disease in the athlete practicing sports with overhead movement.

Halbrecht et al[21] has confirmed via magnetic resonance imaging (MRI) that physical contact of the undersurface of the supraspinatus tendon against the posterior-superior glenoid was found in 10 collegiate baseball pitchers when their pitching arm was placed in the position of 90 degrees of ER and 90 degrees of abduction. Paley et al[22] also published a series on arthroscopic evaluation of the dominant shoulder of 41 professional throwing athletes. With the arthroscope inserted in the glenohumeral joint, they found that 41 out of 41 dominant shoulders evaluated had posterior undersurface impingement between the rotator cuff and posterior superior glenoid. In these professional throwing athletes, 93% had undersurface fraying of the rotator cuff tendons and 88% showed fraying of the posterosuperior glenoid.

### Anterior Internal Impingement

Anterior internal impingement has recently been described as a source of pain in patients with a stable shoulder and positive traditional impingement signs.[23] Struhl[23] reported this phenomenon during arthroscopic evaluation of patients who had clinical signs of traditional outlet impingement and anterior-based pain presentations. Direct visualization during arthroscopy revealed undersurface tears of the rotator cuff due to the contact that occurs between the anterosuperior labrum and undersurface of the rotator cuff, similar to that described by Walch et al[19] in posterior impingement.

In a series of 10 patients with traditional impingement signs and anterior-based pain presentations, Struhl[23] arthroscopically confirmed contact between the fragmented undersurface of the rotator cuff tendons and the anterosuperior labrum during the Hawkins impingement test, viewed from a posterior arthroscopic portal. The understanding of this new clinical entity is essential for both diagnosis and treatment of patients with the clinical appearance of outlet impingement and an anterior pain presentation. It has been hypothesized that shoulder pain seen in swimmers may be the result of anterior internal impingement; the pain is frequently reported at hand entry into the water—in this position, the humeral position is similar to that of the Neer and Hawkins test.[23]

### ◆ Rehabilitation of Rotator Cuff Impingement

It is beyond the scope of this chapter to discuss the complex and comprehensive evaluation methods specifically; however, a detailed and systematic approach to shoulder and upper-extremity evaluation must be undertaken both to identify the specific type of rotator cuff impingement as well as to determine the often-subtle underlying causes. In all types of impingement listed above, scapular dysfunction either can be the underlying cause or can greatly exacerbate the impingement process with altered scapular kinematics in patients with both rotator cuff instability and impingement.[24–26] Initial rehabilitation begins with the protection of the rotator cuff from stress but not function.

### Initial Phase

The rotator cuff must be protected against mechanical compression by the overlying coracoacromial arch or posterior glenoid; this can be done by modifying ergonomic, sport-specific postures and movement patterns as well as those related to activities of daily living (ADL). Modalities such as electrical stimulation, ultrasound, and iontophoresis can be applied to promote improved blood supply and decrease pain levels; however, a clearly superior modality or sequence of modalities for the early management of tendon pathology in the human shoulder is lacking. One study highlights the importance of early submaximal exercise to increase local blood flow. Jensen et al[27] studied the effects of submaximal [5 to 50% maximum voluntary contraction (MVC)] contractions in the supraspinatus tendon measured with laser Doppler flowmetry. Results showed even submaximal contractions increased perfusion during all 1-minute contractions; but they also produced a postcontraction latent hyperemia following the muscular contraction. These findings have provided the rationale for the early use of internal and ER isometrics or submaximal manual resistance in the scapular plane with low levels of elevation to prevent any subacromial contact early in the rehabilitation process.

A key technique in the early management of rotator cuff impingement is scapular stabilization. Manual techniques allow the clinician to interface directly with the patient's scapula to bypass the glenohumeral joint and permit repetitive scapular exercise without inducing undue stress to the rotator cuff in the early

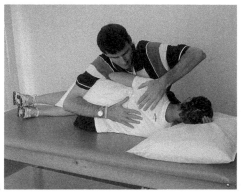
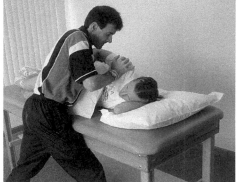

**Figure 1–1(A, B)** Manual scapular stabilization in side-lying position for scapular retraction **(A)**, and protraction **(B)**.

phase. **Figure 1–1A** shows the specific technique I use with my patients to resist scapular retraction manually. Solem-Bertoft et al[28] has shown the importance of scapular retraction posturing by reporting a reduction in the width of the subacromial space when comparing scapular protraction posturing to scapular retraction. Activation of the serratus anterior and lower trapezius force couple is imperative to enable scapular upward rotation and stabilization during arm elevation.[29] Rhythmic stabilization applied to the proximal aspect of the extremity progressing to distal with the glenohumeral joint in 80 to 90 degrees of elevation in the scapular plane (**Fig. 1–2**) can be initiated to provide muscular co-contraction in a functional position. Additionally, with this technique a protracted scapular

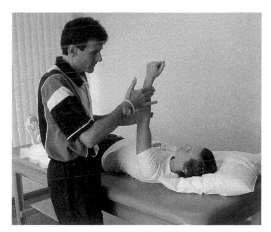

**Figure 1–2** Rhythmic stabilization performed with scapular protraction.

position can be utilized to increase the activation of the serratus anterior muscle[30,31]; several studies have identified decreased muscular activation of this muscle in patients diagnosed with glenohumeral impingement and instability.[25,32]

In addition to the early scapular stabilization and submaximal rotator cuff exercise, ROM and mobilization may be indicated based on the underlying mobility status of the patient. Use of examination procedures to assess the accessory mobility of the glenohumeral joint is of critical importance in guiding this portion of the treatment. Patients with secondary rotator cuff impingement due to underlying instability cannot receive accessory mobilization techniques to increase mobility because this would only compound their existing capsular laxity. However, patients with primary impingement often present with underlying capsular hypomobility and are definite candidates for specific mobilization techniques to improve glenohumeral joint arthrokinematics. One area that has received a great deal of attention in the scientific literature is the presence of an IR ROM limitation, particularly in the overhead athlete with rotator cuff dysfunction.[33,34] To determine the course of treatment for the patient with limited IR ROM, clinical assessment strategies must be employed to determine whether the limitation and subsequent treatment strategy to address the limitation in glenohumeral joint IR should be targeted for the muscle–tendon unit or the posterior capsule.

To determine the tightness of the posterior glenohumeral joint capsule, an accessory mobility technique to assess the mobility of the humeral head relative to the glenoid is recommended. This technique is most often referred to as the *posterior load and shift or posterior drawer test.*[35,36] **Figure 1–3** shows the recommended technique for this examination maneuver whereby the glenohumeral joint is abducted 90 degrees in the scapular plane (note the position of the humerus 30 degrees anterior the coronal plane). The examiner is careful to utilize a posterolaterally directed force (in the direction of the arrow) along the line of the glenohumeral joint. The examiner then feels for translation of the humeral head along the glenoid face. In the grading technique designed by Altchek,[37] grade I is considered normal motion within the glenoid (typically 8 to 10 mm[38]), and a grade II translation is when the clinician-guided stress produces movement of the humeral head over the glenoid rim posteriorly with relocation of the humeral head into the glenoid when stress is removed. Patients presenting with a limitation in IR ROM who have grade II translation should not have posterior glide accessory techniques applied to increase IR ROM due to the hypermobility of the posterior capsule made evident during this important passive clinical test.

It should be pointed out that incorrect use of this posterior glide assessment technique may lead to the false identification of posterior capsular tightness. A common error in this exam technique is the use either of the coronal plane for testing or of a straight posteriorly directed force by the examiner's hand rather than the recommended posterolateral force.

The straight posterior force compresses the humeral head into the glenoid because of the anteverted position of the glenoid; this would inaccurately lead to the assumption by the examining clinician that limited posterior capsular mobility is present.

The second important test to determine the presence of IR ROM limitation is the assessment of physiological ROM. Several authors recommend measurement of glenohumeral IR with the joint in 90 degrees of abduction in the coronal plane.[39–41] During IR ROM measurement (**Fig. 1–4**), care must be taken to stabilize the scapula, with the patient supine so that the patient's body weight can minimize scapular motion as the examiner uses a posteriorly directed force on the anterior aspect of the coracoid and shoulder. Bilateral comparison of IR ROM is taken with careful interpretation of isolated glenohumeral motion.

One rather consistent finding present during the examination of the overhead athlete is increased dominant arm ER as well as reduced dominant arm glenohumeral joint IR.[33,41–43] I have found that this relationship is only identified under conditions where the glenohumeral joint rotation was measured with the scapula stabilized.[44] Failure to stabilize the scapula may not produce glenohumeral joint IR ROM limitations even though they are present, possibly due to scapular compensation. It is important to use consistent measurement techniques when documenting ROM of glenohumeral joint rotation.

Several proposed mechanisms have been discussed attempting to explain this glenohumeral

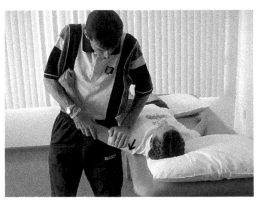

**Figure 1–3** Posterior glenohumeral joint translation test at 90 degrees of abduction in the scapular plane.

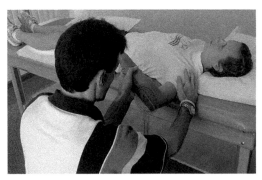

**Figure 1–4** Technique used to measure more isolated glenohumeral joint internal rotation with the shoulder in 90 degrees of abduction in the coronal plane.

ROM relationship of increased ER and limited IR.[33,45,46] The tightness of the posterior capsule as well as the muscle tendon unit of the posterior rotator cuff has been believed to limit internal glenohumeral joint rotation. Additionally, Crockett et al[45] have shown unilateral increases in humeral retroversion in throwing athletes, which would explain the increase in ER with accompanying IR loss. Burkhart et al[34] have termed this IR loss *GIRD–glenohumeral internal rotation deficit*—and define it as a loss of internal rotation of 20 degrees or more compared with the contralateral side.

## Total Rotation Range-of-Motion Concept

To have a numerical representation of the total rotation range of motion available at the glenohumeral joint, the glenohumeral joint IR, and ER ROM measure are added together. Research by Kibler et al[47] and Roetert et al[48] has identified decreases in the total rotation ROM arc in the dominant extremity of elite tennis players correlated with increasing age and number of competitive years of play. Recently, my colleagues and I measured the bilateral total rotation ROM in both professional baseball pitchers and elite junior tennis players.[33] Our findings showed the professional baseball pitchers to have greater dominant arm ER and significantly less dominant arm IR when compared with the contralateral nondominant side. The total rotation ROM, however, was not significantly different between extremities in the professional baseball pitchers (145 degrees dominant arm, 146 degrees nondominant arm). Hence, despite bilateral differences in the actual IR and/or ER ROM in the glenohumeral joints of baseball pitchers, the total arc of rotational motion should remain the same.

In contrast, we tested 117 elite male junior tennis players.[33] In these tennis players, significantly less IR ROM was found on the dominant arm (45 degrees versus 56 degrees), as well as significantly less total rotation ROM on the dominant arm (149 degrees versus 158 degrees). The total rotation ROM did differ between extremities. Approximately 10 degrees less total rotation ROM can be expected in the dominant arm of the uninjured elite junior tennis player as compared with the nondominant extremity.

**Table 1–1** contains the descriptive data from the professional baseball pitchers and elite junior tennis players.[33] More research including additional subject populations is needed to outline the total rotation ROM concept further.

Clinical application of the total rotation ROM concept is best demonstrated by a case presentation of a unilaterally dominant upper-extremity sports athlete. If, during the initial evaluation of a high-level baseball pitcher, the clinician finds a ROM pattern of 120 degrees of ER and only 30 degrees of IR, some uncertainty may exist as to whether that represents a range of motion deficit in IR that requires rehabilitative intervention via stretching and specific mobilization. If measurement of that patient's nondominant extremity rotation, however, reveals 90 degrees of ER and 60 degrees of

**Table 1–1** Bilateral Arm Comparison of Isolated and Total Rotation Range of Motion of Professional Baseball Pitchers and Elite Junior Tennis Players

| Subjects | Dominant Arm (SEM) | Nondominant Arm (SEM) |
| --- | --- | --- |
| **Baseball Pitchers** | | |
| ER | 103.2 ± 9.1 (1.34) | 94.5 ± 8.1 (1.19) |
| IR | 42.4 ± 15.8 (2.33) | 52.4 ± 16.4 (2.42) |
| Total Rotation | 145.6 ± 18.0 (2.66) | 146.9 ± 17.5 (2.59) |
| **Elite Jr. Tennis Players** | | |
| ER | 103.7 ± 10.9 (1.02) | 101.8 ± 10.8 (1.01) |
| IR | 45.4 ± 13.6 (1.28) | 56.3 ± 11.5 (1.08) |
| Total Rotation | 149.1 ± 18.4 (1.73) | 158.1 ± 15.9 (1.50) |

*Note:* All measurements are expressed in degrees.
ER, external rotation; IR, internal rotation; SEM, standard error of the mean.

internal rotation, the current recommendation based on the total rotation ROM concept would be to avoid extensive mobilization and passive stretching of the dominant extremity because the total rotation ROM in both extremities is 150 degrees (120 ER + 30 IR = 150 dominant arm/90 ER and 60 IR = 150 total rotation non-dominant arm). In elite tennis players, the total active rotation ROM can be expected to be up to 10 degrees less on the dominant arm before an extensive clinical treatment to address IR ROM restriction would be recommended or implemented.

This total rotation ROM concept can be used to guide the clinician during rehabilitation, specifically in the application of stretching and mobilization exercises, to best determine what glenohumeral joint requires additional mobility. Equally important is which extremity should not experience additional mobility due to the obvious harm induced by increases in capsular mobility and increases in humeral head translation during aggressive upper-extremity exertion.

The loss of IR ROM is significant for several reasons. The relationship between IR ROM loss (tightness in the posterior capsule of the shoulder) and increased anterior humeral head translation has been identified.[49,50] The increase in anterior humeral shear force reported by Harryman et al[51] was manifested by a horizontal adduction cross-body maneuver, similar to that incurred during the follow-through of the throwing motion or tennis serve. Tightness of the posterior capsule has also been linked to increased superior migration of the humeral head during shoulder elevation.[52]

Koffler et al[53] studied the effects of posterior capsular tightness in a functional position of 90 degrees of abduction and 90 degrees or more of ER in cadaveric specimens. They found, with either imbrication of the inferior aspect of the posterior capsule or imbrication of the entire posterior capsule, that humeral head kinematics were changed or altered. In the presence of posterior capsular tightness, the humeral head will shift in an anterior-superior direction, as compared with a normal shoulder with normal capsular relationships. With more-extensive amounts of posterior capsular tightness, the humeral head was found to shift posterosuperiorly. These effects of altered posterior capsular tension on in vivo posterior glenohumeral joint capsular tightness highlight the clinical importance of utilizing a reliable and effective measurement methodology to assess IR ROM during examination of the shoulder. Additionally, Burkhart et al[34] have clinically demonstrated the concept of posterior-superior humeral head shear in the abducted externally rotated position with tightness of the posterior band of the inferior glenohumeral ligament.

A large spectrum of mobility can be encountered when treating the patient with glenohumeral impingement. Hence, in guiding patients through the rehabilitation process, an accurate ROM measurement and informed decision making are essential to the clinician. To further illustrate the role of ROM and passive stretching during this phase of the rehabilitation, **Figures 1–5** and **1–6** show

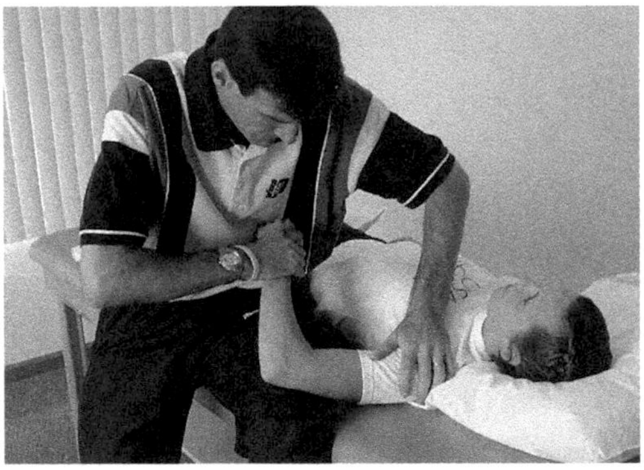

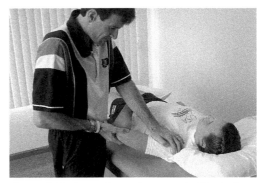

**Figure 1–5** Internal rotation stretch using therapist's leg as a stabilizing platform to allow both hands to control glenohumeral internal rotation and to utilize the scapular plane.

**Figure 1–6** Internal rotation stretch. Hand placements allow for containment of humeral translation and scapular compensation.

versions of clinical IR stretching positions that utilize the scapular plane and can be performed in multiple and varied positions of glenohumeral abduction. Each utilizes an inherent anterior hand placement; this gives varying degrees of posterior pressure to minimize scapular compensation and to provide a check against anterior humeral head translation during the IR stretch. These stretches can be used in a proprioceptive neuromuscular facilitation (PNF) contract–relax format or following a low-load prolonged stretch–type paradigm to facilitate the increase in ROM.[54,55] **Figures 1–7** and **1–8** are examples of home stretches given to patients to address IR ROM deficiency. Note the inherent means of scapular stabilization in both methods that are necessary to optimize the value of the stretching procedure. Recent research has compared the effects of the cross-arm stretch to the sleeper stretch in a population of recreational athletes, some with significant glenohumeral IR range of motion deficiency.[56] Four weeks of stretching produced significantly greater IR gains in the group performing the cross-body stretch as compared with the sleeper stretch. Further research is needed to better define the optimal application of these stretches; however, this research does show improvement in IR ROM with a home stretching program.[56]

At this stage of the rehabilitation program, the clinician should introduce a passive stretching as well as glenohumeral joint mobilization in other directions and movement patterns. Manual assessment of both accessory and physiologic motion guides the clinician in

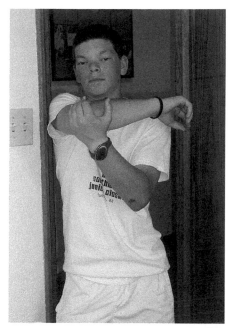

**Figure 1–8** Cross-arm stretch using the wall for additional scapular stabilization to improve internal rotation range of motion.

the application of these interventions to ensure that stretching and mobilization techniques are not performed on a hypermobile joint. By understanding the underlying cause of the rotator cuff dysfunction, the clinician can offset the possibility that joint instability is overlooked in the patient.

Goals in the initial phase of rehabilitation include: (1) to decrease pain to allow for initiation of submaximal rotator cuff and scapular exercise; (2) to normalize capsular relationships using specific mobilization and stretching techniques; and (3) to initiate early submaximal rotator cuff and scapular resistance training.

## Total Arm Strength Phase

The next phase in rehabilitation is dominated by strength and local muscle endurance training of the rotator cuff and scapular stabilizers. Although the entire kinetic chain, including the lower extremity, pelvis, and trunk segments, is also critically important, it is beyond the scope of this chapter to list all kinetic chain exercises indicated. In this section, I will review the use of an evidence-based progression of a

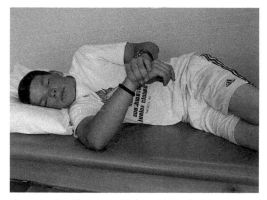

**Figure 1–7** Sleeper stretch used as a home program activity for patients with limited internal rotation range of motion.

resistive exercise program—the primary goals of which are to elicit high levels of rotator cuff and scapular muscular activation using movement patterns and positions that do not create subacromial contact or undue stress to the static stabilizers of the glenohumeral joint. **Figure 1–9** shows the exercise sheet I give my patients, which illustrates the exercises needed for rotator cuff strengthening. These exercises are based on electromyographic (EMG) research showing high levels of posterior rotator cuff activation[57–61]; these movements place the shoulder in positions well tolerated by patients with rotator cuff and scapular dysfunction. A side-lying ER and prone extension exercise with an externally rotated (thumb-out) position is utilized first, with progression to the prone horizontal abduction and prone ER with scapular retraction exercises following a demonstrated tolerance to the initial two exercises. The prone horizontal abduction exercise is used at 90 degrees of abduction to

PERFORM _____ SETS _____ REPS
RESISTANCE LEVEL_____

1. SIDE-LYING EXTERNAL ROTATION:
Lie on uninvolved side, with involved arm at side, with a small pillow between arm and body. Keeping elbow of involved arm bent and fixed to side, raise arm into external rotation. Slowly lower to starting position and repeat.

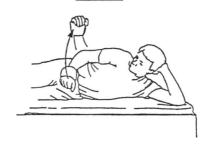

2. SHOULDER EXTENSION:
Lie on table on stomach, with involved arm hanging straight to the floor. With thumb pointed outward, raise arm straight back into extension toward your hip. Slowly lower arm and repeat.

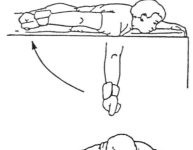

3. PRONE HORIZONTAL ABDUCTION:
Lie on table on stomach, with involved arm hanging straight to the floor. With thumb pointed outward, raise arm out to the side, parallel to the floor. Slowly lower arm, and repeat.

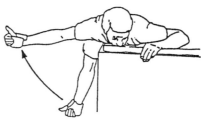

4. 90/90 EXTERNAL ROTATION:
Lie on table on stomach, with shoulder abducted to 90 degrees and arm supported on table, with elbow bent at 90 degrees. Keeping the shoulder and elbow fixed, rotate arm into external rotation, slowly lower to start position, and repeat.

**Figure 1–9**  Rotator cuff exercise progression.

minimize the effects from subacromial contact. Research has shown this position to create high levels of supraspinatus muscular activation,[58,59,61] making it an alternative to the widely used "empty can" exercise, which often can cause impingement due to the combined inherent movements of IR and elevation. Three sets of 15 to 20 repetitions of each exercise are recommended to create a fatigue response. Moncreif et al[62] have demonstrated the efficacy of these exercises in a 4-week training paradigm and measured 8 to 10% increases in isokinetically measured IR and ER strength in healthy subjects. These isotonic exercises are coupled with the ER oscillation exercise (**Fig. 1–10**), which uses 30-second sets and elastic resistance to provide a resistance bias to the posterior rotator cuff.

All exercises for ER strengthening in standing are performed with the addition of a small towel roll placed under the axilla as pictured in **Figure 1–10**. In addition to assisting in the isolation of the exercise and controlling unwanted movements, this towel roll application has been shown to elevate muscular activity by 10% in the infraspinatus muscle when compared with identical exercises performed without the towel placement.[59] Another theoretical advantage of the use of a towel roll to place the shoulder in ~20 to 30 degrees of abduction is to prevent the "wringing out" phenomenon proposed in cadaver-based microvascular research.[63] Rathburn and McNab[63] showed enhanced blood flow in the supraspinatus tendon when the arm was placed in slight abduction as compared with the completely adducted position. Finally, recent research has further supported the use of a towel roll or pillow between the humerus and torso under the axilla during humeral rotational training exercise. Using MRI, Graichen et al[64] studied 12 healthy shoulders at 30, 60, 90, 120, and 150 degrees of abduction. The authors applied a 15 Newton force that resulted in either an abduction isometric contraction or an adduction isometric contraction. The MRI scans showed that adduction isometric muscle contraction produced a significant opening or increase in the subacromial space in all positions of glenohumeral joint abduction. No change in scapular tilting or scapulohumeral rhythm was encountered during the abduction or adduction isometric contractions. Use of the towel roll, therefore, can facilitate an adduction isometric contraction in patients who may need enhanced subacromial intervals during the humeral rotation exercise.[64]

Scapular stabilization exercises are progressed to include ER with retraction (**Fig. 1–11**), an exercise shown to recruit the lower trapezius at a rate 3.3 times more than the upper trapezius and utilize the important position of scapular retraction.[65] Multiple seated-rowing variations, continued manual scapular protraction/retraction, and the use of the 90-degree abducted ER exercise in the prone position (**Fig. 1–9**) are used to facilitate the lower trapezius and other scapular stabilizers[57,66] during this stage of the rehabilitation. Closed chain exercise using the "plus" position that is characterized by maximal scapular protraction has been recommended by Moesley et al[30] and Decker et al[31] for its inherent maximal serratus anterior recruitment. Closed chain step-ups (**Fig. 1–12**), quadruped-position rhythmic stabilization, and variations of the pointer position (**Fig. 1–13**) are all used in endurance-oriented formats (timed sets of 30 seconds) to

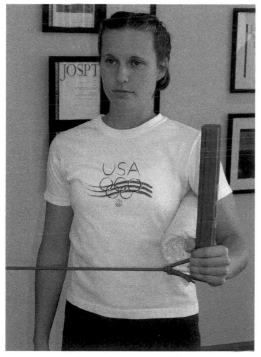

**Figure 1–10** External rotation oscillation.

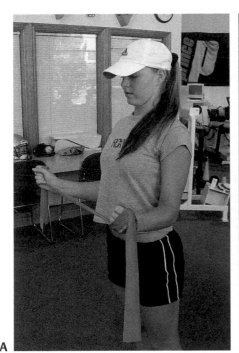
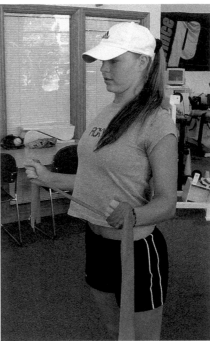

**Figure 1–11(A, B)**  External rotation with retraction exercise. **(A)** Bilateral external rotation performed, **(B)** with superimposed scapular retraction.

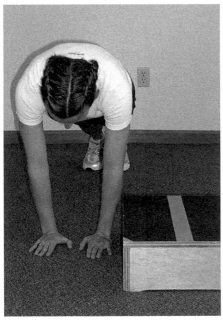
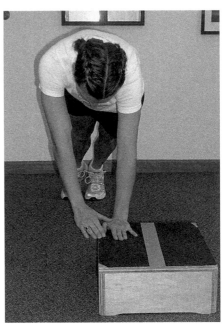

**Figure 1–12(A, B)**  Closed chain step-ups using the "plus" position on the weight-bearing limb: **(A)** start position; **(B)** step-up with involved extremity pressing into the step with scapular protraction.

enhance scapular stabilization. Uhl et al[67] has demonstrated the effects of increasing weight-bearing and successive decreases in the number of weight-bearing limbs on muscle activation of the rotator cuff and scapular musculature. The authors also provide guidance to closed chain exercise progression in the upper extremity.[67]

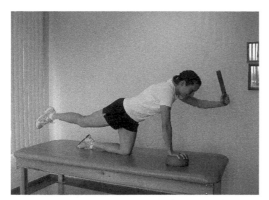

**Figure 1–13** Pointer exercise with medicine ball and oscillation device using the "plus" position on the weight-bearing limb.

Progression to the functional position of 90 degrees of abduction in the scapular plane to simulate the throwing and overhead patterning inherent in many sports activities and daily functions is based on the tolerance of the initial rotator cuff and scapular exercise progression. Bassett et al[68] have shown the importance of training the muscle in the position of function based on the change in muscular lever arms and subsequent function in the 90/90 position. Rhythmic stabilization on a ball (**Fig. 1–14**) is one example of an early abducted exercise with therapist guidance. The scapular plane position is an optimal position for this exercise and other exercises in lower planes of elevation in the earlier phase of rehabilitation as well with humeral elevation to 90 degrees for several important reasons. The inherent optimal bony congruency between the humeral head and glenoid[69]

together with the finding that the rotator cuff is best able to maintain glenohumeral stability with a position of 29.3 degrees makes the scapular plane position an optimal position for rehabilitative exercise.[70]

Additional applications of the 90/90 position include the external oscillation or "Statue of Liberty" exercise (**Fig. 1–15**) and use of the Inertial Exercise Trainer (Impulse Training Systems, Newnan, GA) to provide ER training in a position of scapular retraction. ER fatigue resistance training affects the proper biomechanical function of the entire upper-extremity kinetic chain. Tsai et al[71] demonstrated significant scapular positional changes during the early and middle phases of arm elevation, specifically decreases in posterior scapular tilting and scapular ER following fatigue of the glenohumeral external rotators. This is just one evidence-based rationale for the heavy use of ER-based training for the patient with glenohumeral impingement.

As the patient tolerates isotonic exercise with 2 to 3 pounds and can perform rotational training with medium-level elastic resistance, isokinetic rotational exercise is initiated in the modified-base position. This position places the glenohumeral joint in 30 degrees of flexion,

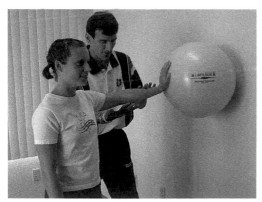

**Figure 1–14** Ninety-degree abducted rhythmic stabilization against an exercise ball in the scapular plane.

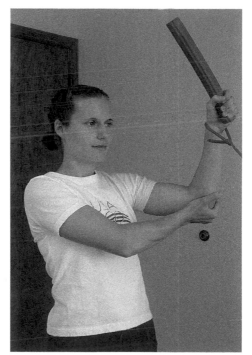

**Figure 1–15** The "Statue of Liberty" exercise.

30 degrees of abduction, and uses a 30-degree tilt of the dynamometer relative to the horizontal (**Fig. 1–16**).[72] This position is well tolerated and allows the patient to progress from submaximal to more maximal levels of resistance at velocities ranging between 120 and 210 deg/s for nonathletic patient populations and between 210 and 360 deg/s during later stages of rehabilitation in more athletic patients. The use of the isokinetic dynamometer is also important to quantify objectively muscular strength levels and, most critically, muscular balance between the internal and external rotators.[73] A goal of achieving a level of IR and ER strength equal to the contralateral extremity is an acceptable initial goal for many patients; however, unilateral increases in IR strength by 15 to 30% have been reported in many descriptive studies of overhead athletes,[42,74–76] and thus may require greater rehabilitative emphasis to achieve this level of documented "dominance."

There is a predominance of IR/ER patterning during isokinetic training. This focus is based on an isokinetic training study by Quincy et al,[77] who showed IR/ER training for a period of 6 weeks to produce not only statistically significant gains in IR and ER strength, but also improved shoulder extension/flexion and abduction/adduction strength as well. Training in the patterns of flexion/extension and abduction/adduction for the same 6 weeks produced only strength gains specific to the direction of training. The more extensive training allows for a more time-efficient and effective focus in the clinic during isokinetic training.

Muscular balance indicated by the ER:IR ratio provides objective information for the clinician to ensure that proper balance between the anterior and posterior dynamic stabilizers is present. Ratios in normal, healthy shoulders have been reported as 66%.[72,73,78] The emphasis on development of the external rotators (posterior rotator cuff) in rehabilitation for anterior instability has led to the concept of a "posterior dominant" shoulder, a shoulder that essentially has a unilateral strength ratio greater than 66% with a goal of 75 to 80% being sought.[73] Careful monitoring through the use of a dynamometer to measure muscular strength allows the clinician to specifically monitor and focus the rehabilitation program to promote the return of muscular balance.

During the end stage of impingement rehabilitation, individuals returning to overhead activities and sports are candidates for advanced isokinetic training using functionally specific rotational training at 90 degrees of abduction in the scapular plane (**Fig. 1–17**) and a plyometric exercise progression. Several studies in the literature do show increases in upper-extremity function with plyometric exercise variations.[79,80] The functional application of the eccentric prestretch followed by a powerful concentric muscular contraction closely parallels many upper-extremity sport activities and makes an excellent exercise modality to transition the active patient to the interval-based sport-return programs described in chapter 9. **Figure 1–18** shows a prone 90/90-position plyometric exercise that can be used with the athlete maintaining a retracted scapular position with the shoulder in 90 degrees of abduction and 90 degrees of ER. The plyometric exercise (plyo) ball is rapidly dropped and caught over a 3- to 5-inch movement distance for sets of 30 to as much as 40 seconds to address local muscular

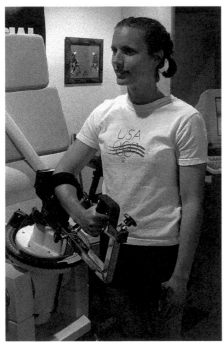

**Figure 1–16** Modified-base position used for initial isokinetic internal/external rotation training and testing.

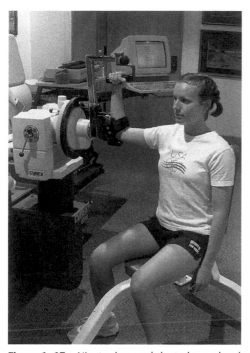

**Figure 1–17** Ninety-degree abducted scapular plane training position

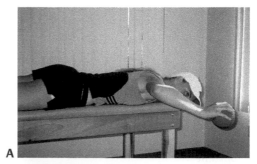

A

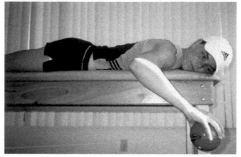

B

**Figure 1–18 (A, B)** Prone 90/90-position (90 degrees of abduction and 90 degrees of external rotation) plyometric exercise for posterior rotator cuff and scapular training.

endurance.[81] **Figure 1–19** shows a reverse catch plyometric exercise that is performed again with the glenohumeral joint in the 90/90 position. The ball is tossed from behind the patient to load eccentrically the posterior rotator cuff (external rotators) with a rapid concentric ER movement performed as the patient throws the ball back while keeping the abducted position of the shoulder along with 90 degrees of elbow flexion. These one-arm plyometric exercises can be preceded by two-arm catches over the shoulder to determine

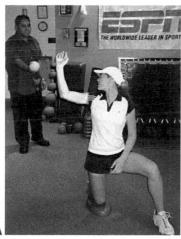

A

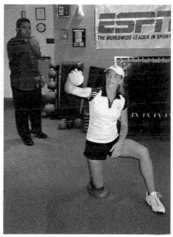

B

**Figure 1–19 (A, B)** Unilateral posterior rotator cuff plyometric exercise simulating the deceleration phase of the throwing or serving motion.

readiness for the one-arm loading. Small half-pound medicine balls or soft weights (Theraband–Hygenic Corp., Akron, OH) are used initially with progression to 1 to 2 pounds as the patient progresses in both skill and strength development. **Figures 1–20** and **1–21** show closed chain exercises using plyo balls that are used to encourage scapular stabilization. The use of heavy loading is avoided throughout rehabilitation due to the likely unwanted muscular compensation and use of superior scapular positioning and "shrugging" during the performance of overloaded upper-extremity exercise.

### Discharge Considerations

A multifaceted approach is recommended when determining when the patient is ready for progression to an interval-based sport-return program (see chapter 9), and ultimately considered for discharge from formal physical therapy. Areas for consideration are normalization of previously positive manual special tests, ROM, strength, and functional status.

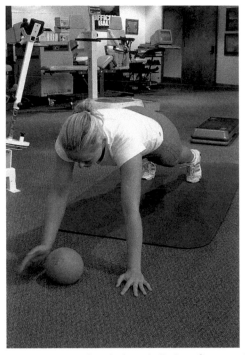

**Figure 1–20** Closed chain ball slaps for scapular stabilization.

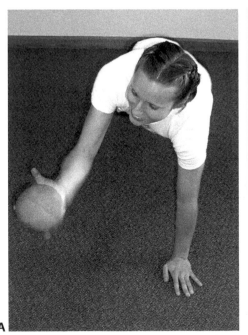
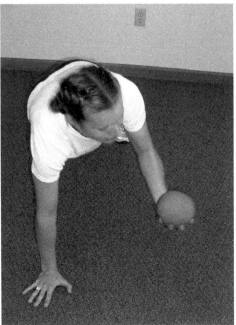

A                   B

**Figure 1–21 (A, B)** Closed chain quadruped alternating unilateral ball catches.

The use of manual orthopaedic tests to diagnose the patient with glenohumeral impingement should be revisited and ultimately be negative to consider progression to advanced activities and discharge.[36] The negative traditional impingement tests of Neer,[2] Hawkins,[82] and Yocum,[84] as well as the cross-arm test,[83] all compromise the subacromial space using specific movement patterns encountered during ADL and functional activities and can give valuable insight into the patient's ability to tolerate these functional positions. Additionally, provocation tests such as the subluxation/relocation test[85] can be very important to determine the patient's competency and stability in the abducted, externally rotated position.[36]

Evaluation of glenohumeral joint ROM is another important discharge parameter. A premature return of the patient to overhead throwing activity with significant ER ROM limitation may further compromise shoulder function as well as distal elbow loading.[86] As has been described in this chapter, normalization of the glenohumeral capsular relationships resulting in a restoration of optimal glenohumeral IR and ER ROM is of critical importance.

Additionally, an evaluation of muscular strength is of critical importance in discharge planning. While an isokinetic or computerized device cannot always be available in all settings and applications, the use of manual muscle testing to determine bilateral symmetry of the key components of the deltoid rotator cuff force couple[87,88] and scapular stabilizers[89] is warranted. In many applications, significantly greater dominant arm strength can be expected and worked toward prior to the return of overhead athletic function.[74–76] The ER:IR unilateral strength ratio is emphasized in my discharge planning because of the importance of muscular balance and optimal posterior rotator cuff stabilization required for pain-free shoulder function. Ratios of 66 to 75% are targeted and can be measured with either isokinetic or isometric dynamometry.[73]

Finally, the functional indexes or rating scales are used to include the patient's perception of shoulder function in the clinical decision-making process. Commonly used rating scales such as the American Shoulder Elbow Surgeons' (ASES), University of California–Los Angeles' (UCLA), and Rowe scales are used in athletic populations and provide valuable information regarding the patient's perception of function.[90,91] The numeric nature of these scales provides longitudinal comparison if used throughout the rehabilitation process or comparison to normative levels.[36,90,91]

### ◆ Outcomes

The final point of discussion in this chapter involves the degree of success or the outcome of nonoperative treatment for shoulder impingement. One of the largest nonoperative studies of shoulder impingement was performed by Morrison et al.[92] They reported on a series of 636 shoulders diagnosed with subacromial impingement. Nonoperative treatment consisting of physical therapy and nonsteroidal antiinflammatory medication resulted in successful resolution of patient symptoms in 67% (426) of the 636 cases. Success, however, was further analyzed and was found to be related to the patient's acromial type. Nonoperative treatment was 91% successful in patients with a type I acromion, 68% for patients with a type II acromion, and 64% successful in patients with a type III or hooked acromion. Additionally, a 78% success rate was reported when the symptoms of subacromial impingement were present for 4 weeks or less prior to the initiation of treatment, whereas only 63% success was found when the symptoms were present for >1 month.

Another study of subacromial impingement demonstrates the effectiveness of resistive exercise to promote muscular balance and in particular to strengthen the humeral head depressors. Walther et al[93] studied 60 patients diagnosed with subacromial impingement and placed 20 patients each into a conventional physical therapy group, a guided home exercise group, and a control group whose members all wore a brace. Constant-Murley scores[95] were assessed at 6 and 12 weeks following initiation of the treatment, with all three groups showing significant improvement. Of particular interest was the finding of improved functional rating scores in the two groups treated with resistive exercises to improve the strength of the humeral head depressors and scapular stabilizers. This study supports the use of targeted resistive exercise in the treatment of subacromial impingement. It is unknown why the subjects wearing the brace improved in this study.

Finally, one question often asked by patients diagnosed with subacromial impingement is whether they would require surgery for complete resolution of their symptoms and how surgical treatment might compare with nonoperative physical therapy. Haahr et al[94] used a prospective randomized research design to study the effects of exercise-based rehabilitation in physical therapy with arthroscopic subacromial decompression in 96 patients aged 18 to 55. Outcome was assessed using the Constant-Murley rating scale and a pain and dysfunction score at 12 months. Results showed significant improvements in both groups from baseline values regardless of whether the patient had surgery or physical therapy. No significant difference existed in the level of improvement between surgery and therapy for the treatment of subacromial impingement. This study supports nonoperative physical therapy as a viable treatment for the patient with subacromial impingement.

## ◆ Summary

A detailed clinical examination and evidence-based rehabilitation program focusing on restoring normal glenohumeral joint arthrokinematics and improving rotator cuff strength and scapular stabilization are important factors in the treatment of the patient with shoulder impingement. Recognition of the many types of impingement as well as an understanding of the underlying cause of the impingement process are of paramount importance in the development of effective treatment strategies to restore full function in patients with this dysfunction.

## References

1. Neer CS 2nd. Anterior acromioplasty for the chronic impingement syndrome in the shoulder: a preliminary report. J Bone Joint Surg Am 1972;54:41–50
2. Neer CS 2nd. Impingement lesions. Clin Orthop Relat Res 1983;173:70–77
3. Golding FC. The shoulder: the forgotten joint. Br J Radiol 1962;35:149–158
4. Cotton RE, Rideout DF. Tears of the humeral rotator cuff: a radiological and pathological necropsy survey. J Bone Joint Surg Br 1964;46:314–328
5. Flatow EL, Soslowsky LJ, Ticker JB, et al. Excursion of the rotator cuff under the acromion: patterns of subacromial contact. Am J Sports Med 1994;22: 779–788
6. Poppen NK, Walker PS. Forces at the glenohumeral joint in abduction. Clin Orthop Relat Res 1978;135: 165–170
7. Lucas DB. Biomechanics of the shoulder joint. Arch Surg 1973;107:425–432
8. Wuelker N, Plitz W, Roetman B. Biomechanical data concerning the shoulder impingement syndrome. Clin Orthop Relat Res 1994;303:242–249
9. Fleisig GS, Andrews JR, Dillman CJ, Escamilla RF. Kinetics of baseball pitching with implications about injury mechanisms. Am J Sports Med 1995;23: 233–239
10. Elliott B, Marsh T, Blanksby B. A three dimensional cinematographic analysis of the tennis serve. Int J Sport Biomechanics 1986;2:260–271
11. Bigliani LU, Ticker JB, Flatow EL, et al. The relationship of acromial architecture to rotator cuff disease. Clin Sports Med 1991;10:823–838
12. Zuckerman JD, Kummer FJ, Cuomo F, et al. The influence of coracoacromial arch anatomy on rotator cuff tears. J Shoulder Elbow Surg 1992;1:4–14
13. Jobe FW, Kivitne RS. Shoulder pain in the overhand or throwing athlete. Orthop Rev 1989;18:963–975
14. Andrews JR, Alexander EJ. Rotator cuff injury in throwing and racquet sports. Sports Med Arthroscopy Rev 1995;3:30–38
15. Wilk KE, Arrigo CA. Current concepts in the rehabilitation of the athletic shoulder. J Orthop Sports Phys Ther 1993;18:365–378
16. Ellenbecker TS. Rehabilitation of shoulder and elbow injuries in tennis players. Clin Sports Med 1995; 14:87–110
17. Nirschl RP. Shoulder tendonitis. In: Pettrone FA, ed. Upper Extremity Injuries in Athletes. Proceedings of the American Academy of Orthopaedic Surgeons Symposium. Philadelphia, PA: Mosby; 1986 pp. 332–337
18. Jobe FW, Pink M. The athlete's shoulder. J Hand Ther 1994;7:107–110
19. Walch G, Boileau P, Noel E, Donell ST. Impingement of the deep surface of the supraspinatus tendon on the posterosuperior glenoid rim: an arthroscopic study. J Shoulder Elbow Surg 1992;1:238–245
20. Gerber C, Galantay RV, Hersche O. The pattern of pain produced by irritation of the acromioclavicular joint and the subacromial space. J Shoulder Elbow Surg 1998;7:352–355
21. Halbrecht JL, Tirman P, Atkin D. Internal impingement of the shoulder: comparison of findings between the throwing and nonthrowing shoulders of college baseball players. Arthroscopy 1999;15:253–258
22. Paley KJ, Jobe FW, Pink MM, Kvitne RS, ElAttarche NS. Arthroscopic findings in the overhand throwing athlete: evidence for posterior internal impingement of the rotator cuff. Arthroscopy 2000;16:35–40
23. Struhl S. Anterior internal impingement: an arthroscopic observation. Arthroscopy 2002;18:2–7
24. Warner JJ, Micheli LJ, Arslanian LE, Kennedy J, Kennedy R. Scapulothoracic motion in normal shoulders and shoulders with glenohumeral instability and impingement syndrome: a study using moire topographic analysis. Clin Orthop Relat Res 1992; 285:191–199

25. Ludewig PM, Cook TM. Alternations in shoulder kinematics and associated muscle activity in people with symptoms of shoulder impingement. Phys Ther 2000;80:276–291

26. Kibler WB. The role of the scapula in athletic shoulder function. Am J Sports Med 1998;26:325–337

27. Jensen BR, Sjogaard G, Bornmyr S, Arborelius M, Jorgensen K. Intramuscular laser-Doppler flowmetry in the supraspinatus muscle during isometric contractions. Eur J Appl Physiol Occup Physiol 1995;71:373–378

28. Solem-Bertoft E, Thuomas KA, Westerberg CE. The influence of scapula retraction and protraction on the width of the subacromial space. An MRI study. Clin Orthop Relat Res 1993;296:99–103

29. Bagg SD, Forrest WJ. A biomechanical analysis of scapular rotation during arm abduction in the scapular plane. Am J Phys Med Rehabil 1988;67:238–245

30. Moseley JB Jr, Jobe FW, Pink M, Perry J, Tibone J. EMG analysis of the scapular muscles during a shoulder rehabilitation program. Am J Sports Med 1992;20:128–134

31. Decker MJ, Hintermeister RA, Faber KJ, Hawkins RJ. Serratus anterior muscle activity during selected rehabilitation exercises. Am J Sports Med 1999;27:784–791

32. McMahon PJ, Jobe FW, Pink MM, Brault JR, Perry J. Comparative electromyographic analysis of shoulder muscles during planar motions: anterior glenohumeral instability versus normal. J Shoulder Elbow Surg 1996;5:118–123

33. Ellenbecker TS, Roetert EP, Bailie DS, Davies GJ, Brown SW. Glenohumeral joint total rotation range of motion in elite tennis players and baseball pitchers. Med Sci Sports Exerc 2002;34:2052–2056

34. Burkhart SS, Morgan CD, Kibler WB. The disabled throwing shoulder: spectrum of pathology, I: pathoanatomy and biomechanics. Arthroscopy 2003;19:404–420

35. McFarland EG, Torpey BM, Carl LA. Evaluation of shoulder laxity. Sports Med 1996;22:264–272

36. Ellenbecker TS. Clinical Examination of the Shoulder. Philadelphia, PA: Elsevier Saunders; 2004

37. Altchek DW, Dines DW. The surgical treatment of anterior instability: selective capsular repair. Op Tech Sports Med 1993;1:285–292

38. Harryman DT 2nd, Sidles JA, Harris SL, Matsen FA. Laxity of the normal glenohumeral joint: in-vivo assessment. J Shoulder Elbow Surg 1992;1:66–76

39. Awan R, Smith J, Boon AJ. Measuring shoulder internal rotation range of motion: a comparison of 3 techniques. Arch Phys Med Rehabil 2002;83:1229–1234

40. Boon AJ, Smith J. Manual scapular stabilization: its effect on shoulder rotational range of motion. Arch Phys Med Rehabil 2000;81:978–983

41. Ellenbecker TS, Roetert EP, Piorkowski PA, Schulz DA. Glenohumeral joint internal and external rotation range of motion in elite junior tennis players. J Orthop Sports Phys Ther 1996;24:336–341

42. Ellenbecker TS. Shoulder internal and external rotation strength and range of motion in highly skilled tennis players. Isok Exercise Science 1992;2:1–8

43. Brown LP, Neihues SL, Harrah A, et al. Upper extremity range of motion and isokinetic strength of the internal and external shoulder rotators in major league baseball players. Am J Sports Med 1988;16:577–585

44. Ellenbecker TS, Roetert EP, Piorkowski PA. Shoulder internal and external rotation range of motion of elite junior tennis players: a comparison of two protocols. J Orthop Sports Phys Ther 1993;17:65 (Abstract)

45. Crockett HC, Gross LB, Wilk KE, et al. Osseous adaptation and range of motion at the glenohumeral joint in professional baseball pitchers. Am J Sports Med 2002;30:20–26

46. Meister K, Day T, Horodyski MB, Kaminski TW, Wasik MP, Tillman S. Rotational motion changes in the glenohumeral joint of the adolescent little league baseball player. Am J Sports Med 2005;33:693–698

47. Kibler WB, Chandler TJ, Livingston BP, Roetert EP. Shoulder range of motion in elite tennis players. Am J Sports Med 1996;24:279–285

48. Roetert EP, Ellenbecker TS, Brown SW. Shoulder internal and external rotation range of motion in nationally ranked junior tennis players: a longitudinal analysis. J Strength Cond Res 2000;14:140–143

49. Tyler TF, Nicholas SJ, Roy T, Gleim GW. Quantification of posterior capsular tightness and motion loss in patients with shoulder impingement. Am J Sports Med 2000;28:668–673

50. Gerber C, Werner CM, Macy JC, Jacob HA, Nyffeller RW. Effect of selective capsulorraphy on the passive range of motion of the glenohumeral joint. J Bone Joint Surg Am 2003;85-A:48–55

51. Harryman DT 2nd, Sidles JA, Clark MJ, McQuade KK, Gibb TD, Matsen FA 3rd. Translation of the humeral head on the glenoid with passive glenohumeral motion. J Bone Joint Surg Am 1990;72:1334–1343

52. Matsen FA III, Artnz CT. Subacromial impingement. In: Rockwood CA Jr, Matsen FA III, eds. The Shoulder. Philadelphia, PA: WB Saunders; 1990 pp. 623–636

53. Koffler KM, Bader D, Eager M, Moyer R, Kely JD. The effect of posterior capsular tightness on glenohumeral translation in the late-cocking phase of pitching: a cadaveric study. Abstract (SS-15) presented at Arthroscopy Association of North America Annual Meeting, Washington, DC, 2001

54. Sullivan PE, Markos PD, Minor MD. An Integrated Approach to Therapeutic Exercise: Theory and Clinical Application. Reston, VA: Reston Publishing; 1982

55. Zachezwski JE, Reischl S. Flexibility for the runner: specific program considerations. Topics in Acute Care and Trauma Rehabilitation 1986;1:9–27

56. McClure P, Balaicuis J, Heiland D, Richard ME, Thorndike C, Wood A. A randomized controlled comparison of stretching procedures in recreational athletes with posterior shoulder tightness [abstract]. J Orthop Sports Phys Ther 2005;35:A5

57. Ballantyne BT, O'Hare SJ, Paschall JL, et al. Electromyographic activity of selected shoulder muscles in commonly used therapeutic exercises. Phys Ther 1993;73:668–682

58. Blackburn TA, McLeod WD, White B, et al. EMG analysis of posterior rotator cuff exercises. Athletic Training 1990;25:40

59. Reinold MM, Wilk KE, Fleisig GS, et al. Electromyographic analysis of the rotator cuff and deltoid musculature during common shoulder external rotation exercises. J Orthop Sports Phys Ther 2004;34:385–394

60. Townsend H, Jobe FW, Pink M, et al. Electromyographic analysis of the glenohumeral muscles

during a baseball rehabilitation program. Am J Sports Med 1991;19:264–272

61. Malanga GA, Jenp YN, Growney ES, An KN. EMG analysis of shoulder positioning in testing and strengthening the supraspinatus. Med Sci Sports Exerc 1996;28:661–664

62. Moncrief SA, Lau JD, Gale JR, Scott SA. Effect of rotator cuff exercise on humeral rotation torque in healthy individuals. J Strength Cond Res 2002;16:262–270

63. Rathbun JB, MacNab I. The microvascular pattern of the rotator cuff. J Bone Joint Surg Br 1970;52:540–553

64. Graichen H, Hinterwimmer S, von Eisenhart-Roth RVR, Vogl T, Englmeier KH, Eckstein F. Effect of abducting and adducting muscle activity on gleno-humeral translation, scapular kinematics and sub-acromial space width in vivo. J Biomech 2005;38:755–760

65. McCabe RA, Tyler TF, Nicholas SJ, McHugh MP. Selective activation of the lower trapezius muscle in patients with shoulder impingement [abstract]. J Orthop Sports Phys Ther 2001;31:A-45

66. Englestad ED, Johnson RL, Jeno SHN, Mabey RL. An electromyographical study of lower trapezius muscle activity during exercise in traditional and modified positions [abstract]. J Orthop Sports Phys Ther 2001;31:A-29–A-30

67. Uhl TL, Carver TJ, Mattacola CG, Mair SD, Nitz AJ. Shoulder musculature activation during upper extremity weightbearing exercise. J Orthop Sports Phys Ther 2003;33:109–117

68. Bassett RW, Browne AO, Morrey BF, An KN. Glenohumeral muscle force and moment mechanics in a position of shoulder instability. J Biomech 1990;23:405–415

69. Saha AK. Mechanism of shoulder movements and a plea for the recognition of "zero position" of glenohumeral joint. Clin Orthop Relat Res 1983;173:3–10

70. Happee R, VanDer Helm CT. The control of shoulder muscles during goal directed movements, an inverse dynamic analysis. J Biomech 1995;28:1179–1191

71. Tsai NT, McClure PW, Karduna AR. Effects of muscle fatigue on 3-dimensional scapular kinematics. Arch Phys Med Rehabil 2003;84:1000–1005

72. Davies GJ. A compendium of isokinetics in clinical usage. LaCrosse, WI: S & S Publishers; 1992

73. Ellenbecker TS, Davies GJ. The application of isokinetics in testing and rehabilitation of the shoulder complex. J Athletic Training 2000;35:338–350

74. Ellenbecker T, Roetert EP. Age specific isokinetic glenohumeral internal and external rotation strength in elite junior tennis players. J Sci Med Sport 2003;6:63–70

75. Ellenbecker TS, Mattalino AJ. Concentric isokinetic shoulder internal and external rotation strength in professional baseball pitchers. J Orthop Sports Phys Ther 1997;25:323–328

76. Wilk KE, Andrews JR, Arrigo CA, Keirns MA, Erber DJ. The strength characteristics of internal and external rotator muscles in professional baseball pitchers. Am J Sports Med 1993;21:61–66

77. Quincy RI, Davies GJ, Kolbeck KJ, Szymanski JL. Isokinetic exercise: the effects of training specificity on shoulder strength development. J Athletic Training 2000;35:S64

78. Ivey FM, Calhoun JH, Rusche K, Bierschenk J. Isokinetic testing of shoulder strength: normal values. Arch Phys Med Rehabil 1985;66:384–386

79. Vossen JE, Kramer JE, Bruke DG, Vossen DP. Comparison of dynamic push-up training and plyo-metric push-up training on upper-body power and strength. J Strength Cond Res 2000;14:248–253

80. Schulte-Edelmann JA, Davies GJ, Kernozek TW, Gerberding ED. The effects of plyometric training of the posterior shoulder and elbow. J Strength Cond Res 2005;19:129–134

81. Fleck SJ, Kraemer WJ. Designing Resistance Training Programs. Champaign IL: Human Kinetics Publishers; 1987

82. Hawkins RJ, Kennedy JC. Impingement syndrome in athletes. Am J Sports Med 1980;8:151–158

83. Davies GJ, DeCarlo MS. Examination of the Shoulder Complex: Current Concepts in Rehabilitation of the Shoulder. Sports Physical Therapy Association Home Study Course. LaCrosse, WI: Sports Physical Therapy Association; 1995

84. Leroux JL, Thomas E, Bonnel F, Blotman F. Diagnostic value of clinical tests for shoulder impingement syndrome. Rev Rhum Engl Ed 1995;62:423–428

85. Hamner DL, Pink MM, Jobe FW. A modification of the relocation test: arthroscopic findings associated with a positive test. J Shoulder Elbow Surg 2000;9:263–267

86. Marshall RN, Elliott BC. Long-axis rotation: the missing link in proximal to distal sequencing. J Sports Sci 2000;18:247–254

87. Inman VT, Saunders JB, Abbott LC. Observations on the function of the shoulder joint. J Bone Joint Surg 1944;26:1–30

88. Kelly BT, Kadrmas WH, Speer KP. The manual muscle examination for rotator cuff strength: an electromyographic investigation. Am J Sports Med 1996;24:581–588

89. Donatelli R, Ellenbecker TS, Ekedahl SR, Wilkes JS, Kocher K, Adam J. Assessment of shoulder strength in professional baseball pitchers. J Orthop Sports Phys Ther 2000;30:544–551

90. Ellenbecker TS, Nazal F, Roetert EP, Bailie DS, Stark R. Shoulder rating scale data from healthy unilaterally dominant overhead sports [abstract]. J Orthop Sports Phys Ther 2005;35:A-79

91. Romeo AA, Bach BR, O'Halloran KL. Scoring systems for shoulder conditions. Am J Sports Med 1996;24:472–476

92. Morrison DS, Frogameni AD, Woodworth P. Non-operative treatment of subacromial impingement syndrome. J Bone Joint Surg Am 1997;79:732–737

93. Walther M, Werner A, Stahlschmidt T, Woelfel R, Gohlke F. The subacromial impingement syndrome of the shoulder treated by conventional physiotherapy, self-training, and a shoulder brace: results of a prospective, randomized study. J Shoulder Elbow Surg 2004;13:417–423

94. Haahr JP, Ostergaard S, Dalsgaard J, et al. Exercises versus arthroscopic decompression in patients with subacromial impingement: a randomized, controlled study in 90 cases with one year follow-up. Ann Rheum Dis 2005;64:760–764

95. Constant CR, Murley AHG. A clinical method of functional assessment of the shoulder. Clin Orthop Rel Research 1987;214:160–164

# 2

# Rehabilitation of Micro-Instability

**Michael M. Reinold, Leonard C. Macrina, Kevin E. Wilk, and James R. Andrews**

Shoulder instability is a common pathology often seen in the orthopaedic and sports medicine setting. The glenohumeral joint requires tremendous amounts of joint mobility to function, thus making it inherently unstable. Due to the significant glenohumeral joint capsular laxity, the differentiation between normal translation and pathological instability is often difficult to determine. Furthermore, a wide range of shoulder instabilities exists, from traumatic dislocations resulting in capsulolabral disruption to repetitive subluxations and multidirectional instability often observed with congenital laxity.

The overhead athlete, however, is unique and typically presents with a certain degree of acquired laxity from the inherent stresses observed during competition. Although necessary to perform at a competitive level, this acquired laxity may progress to excessive micro-instability and lead to pathologies such as rotator cuff and labral degeneration, fraying, or lesions.

In this chapter, our purpose is to overview the classification and mechanism of acquired laxity in overhead athletes, to review common examination techniques used to determine the extent of pathology in these patients, and to discuss the specific rehabilitation principles and guidelines used to treat patients with pathological acquired micro-instability.

## ◆ Presentation and Mechanism of Acquired Laxity

Functional stability of the shoulder is achieved through the precise interaction of the static and dynamic stabilizing systems of the glenohumeral joint. Static stability is accomplished via the joint geometry, capsule, glenohumeral ligaments, and labrum. Because of the required amount of motion of the shoulder, particularly in the overhead athlete, static stability is often compromised, demanding a greater amount of dynamic stability to remain asymptomatic.

Dynamic stability is achieved through the precise neuromuscular interaction of the force couples of the rotator cuff and the shoulder musculature.[34,36] The need for excessive motion in the shoulder of overhead athletes requires the dynamic stabilizers to perform efficiently, particularly near end range of motion (ROM) when static stability is most compromised.

Most overhead athletes exhibit significant laxity of the glenohumeral joint. This allows them to accomplish the necessary motions required to perform their sport. One significant difference between overhead athletes and nonoverhead athletes is shoulder ROM. The typical overhead athlete exhibits excessive external rotation (ER) and decreased internal rotation (IR) at 90 degrees abduction in the throwing shoulder.[4,5,13,35] Brown et al[5] reported that the mean ROM in 41 professional baseball pitchers was 141 degrees ± 15 degrees of shoulder ER at 90 degrees abduction and 83 degrees ± 14 degrees of IR. External rotation was 9 degrees greater in the throwing shoulder than in the nonthrowing shoulder, whereas IR was 15 degrees less than in the nonthrowing shoulder. Furthermore, ER of the throwing shoulder was 9 degrees greater in pitchers than in positional players. Similarly, Bigliani et al[4] evaluated the ROM characteristics in 148 professional baseball players. The authors reported a mean of 118 degrees ER at 90 degrees abduction (range 95 to 145 degrees) in the throwing shoulder of pitchers and a mean of 108 degrees ER in positional players. A statistically significant increase in ER and decrease in IR was observed between the dominant and nondominant shoulder.

Wilk et al[36] reported the shoulder ROM characteristics in 372 professional baseball players. The authors reported a mean of 129 degrees ± 10 degrees of ER and 61 degrees ± 9 degrees of IR in the throwing shoulder at 90 degrees abduction. The authors noted that ER was 7 degrees greater and IR was 7 degrees less in the dominant arm when compared with the nondominant arm. Wilk et al[36] introduced the concept of "total motion," and defined it as the sum of ER and IR at 90 degrees abduction (**Fig. 2–1**). The authors noted that total motion is equal bilaterally in most throwers, usually within 7 degrees. These findings were similar to those reported by Ellenbecker et al[9] in a group of tennis players.

There are several theories explaining why the overhead athlete presents with these unique ROM characteristics. The repetitive microtraumatic stresses placed on the athlete's shoulder joint complex during the throwing motion challenges the physiologic limits of the surrounding tissues. During the overhead throwing motion, the athlete places excessive stresses at the end ROM while generating tremendous angular velocities. Fleisig et al[10]

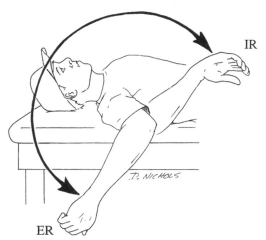

**Figure 2–1** Total motion concept in the overhead athlete. (From Wilk KE, Meister K, Andrews JR. Current concepts in the rehabilitation of the overhead throwing athlete. Am J Sports Med 2002;30:137 Figure 1. Reprinted with permission.)

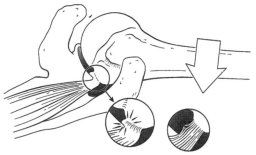

**Figure 2–2** Internal impingement leading to degeneration of the under surface of the rotator cuff. (From Walch G, Boileau P, Noel E, et al. Impingement of the deep surface of the supraspinatus tendon on the posterosuperior glenoid rim: an arthroscopic study. J Shoulder Elbow Surg 1992;1:243, Figure 5A. Reprinted with permission.)

have reported the angular velocity of the arm during the overhead throw to reach 7265 deg/s, which is the fastest human movement. Furthermore, these forces are generated when the shoulder joint is at end range ER, often at 145 to 165 degrees of ER. This results in high forces generated and dissipated at the joint and the supporting structures (i.e., capsule and/or musculature).[39] Fleisig et al[10] reported anterior forces up to $1^1/_2$ times body weight during ER (late cocking) and up to one and one-half times body weight distracting the joint during the follow-through phase. Consequently, the overhead athlete often presents with acquired anterior laxity due to the stresses placed on the joint throughout the throwing motion. Thus, the shoulder complex greatly relies on the dynamic stabilizers because of the compromised static stability often present.

Previous authors have hypothesized that the loss of IR ROM can be attributed to posterior capsular contraction.[6] However, this has been disputed by evidence of osseous retroversion of the humerus[8,19,21] as well as excessive posterior laxity even in patients with marked loss of IR.

Furthermore, Reinold et al[24] recently noted that ROM is affected by overhead throwing. The authors evaluated shoulder ROM in 31 professional baseball pitchers before and immediately after baseball pitching. External rotation before throwing (133 degrees ± 11 degrees) did

not significantly change after throwing (131 degrees ± 10 degrees). However, there was a statistically significant decrease in IR ROM after pitching (73 degrees ± 16 degrees before, 65 degrees ± 11 degrees after) and a subsequent decrease of 9 degrees of total motion. The authors hypothesized that this decrease in IR ROM was due to the large eccentric forces observed in the external rotators during the follow-through phase of throwing.

Thus, it appears that the ROM characteristics of the overhead athlete are due to a combination of factors, including acquired laxity of the anterior capsule, soft tissue adaptations of the posterior rotator cuff, and osseous adaptations of the humerus.

Because of the delicate balance between acquired laxity and pathological micro-instability, the overhead athlete is continuously challenged to perform efficiently and remain asymptomatic. When the overhead athlete develops excessive laxity in the shoulder, it is most often a pathological micro-instability rather than gross macro-instability.

The excessive amounts of translation observed in the athlete with acquired laxity may lead to several pathological conditions such as SLAP (superior labrum anteroposterior) lesions[2] and impingement of the undersurface of the infraspinatus on the posterosuperior labrum.[28] This is referred to as *internal impingement* and may lead to degeneration of the undersurface of the rotator cuff and labrum (**Fig. 2–2**). The phenomenon of internal impingement is one of the most common diagnoses observed in the overhead athlete.

## Common Examination Techniques

A thorough evaluation of the shoulder, including clearing examinations of the proximal and distal segments, is required to appreciate the nature and extent of the pathology. Examination techniques are performed to assess active and passive ROM, laxity, and muscle strength. The examiner may also perform several special tests to assess the integrity of the rotator cuff, labrum, and capsule. Although necessary to perform a complete and thorough evaluation, this is beyond our scope here; other authors review these tests and techniques in later chapters. We will briefly review a few tests that we feel are specific to the patient with micro-instability. The focus of the examination of these patients is the ROM characteristics and the capsular tissue laxity to determine the extent of instability.

As discussed previously, total motion should be equal bilaterally. Total motion is routinely assessed clinically by simply adding ER and IR ROM using standard goniometric measurements. Athletes with symptomatic complaints of micro-instability will often present with a decrease in total motion when compared bilaterally. This overall loss of total motion is often attributed to loss of IR rather than ER. Theoretically, we believe that the loss of IR in the symptomatic athlete can be attributed to pathology of the posterior rotator cuff (rather than posterior capsule), resulting in fibrosis and loss of IR motion.

Several tests may be performed to assess laxity of the capsular tissue. We commonly perform the sulcus sign, anterior and posterior drawers, and the anterior fulcrum tests.

A simple technique used to determine generalized laxity of the glenohumeral joint is the sulcus maneuver.[17,26] The sulcus sign is designed to assess inferior laxity and may be performed at various degrees of abduction. We routinely perform the test in the seated position at 0 degrees of abduction, which assesses the coracohumeral ligament and superior glenohumeral ligament.[29] The test is performed by providing long-axis distraction of the humerus while grasping the bicondylar axis of the humerus and palpating the lateral subacromial space (**Fig. 2–3**). Normal motion varies between 5 and 15 mm depending on the patient population being assessed.[12,14] We feel

that a positive sulcus sign is present when there is greater than 10 mm of inferior humeral translation. This represents a degree of congenital laxity that may be present; we use it to determine the progress rate of our rehabilitation program. Individuals with significant congenital laxity (as indicated by a positive sulcus sign) may be progressed more slowly with specific emphasis on enhancing dynamic stability.

The examiner performs specific techniques to assess anterior[3] and posterior laxity.[11] The anterior and posterior drawer tests are performed with the patient supine. The examiner grasps the arm at the bicondylar axis of the distal humerus. The patient's arm is held in the scapular plane with neutral rotation. The proximal hand grasps the humeral head, which is gently compressed, then translated anteriorly or posteriorly. The tests can be performed at various degrees of shoulder abduction to assess the integrity of specific capsular ligaments (**Fig. 2–4**).

Another test commonly performed for overhead athletes with micro-instability is the anterior fulcrum test. This test is performed

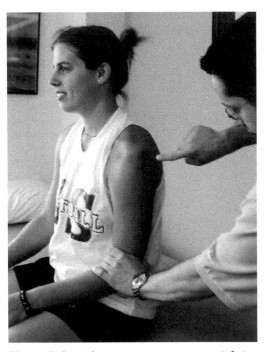

**Figure 2–3** Sulcus maneuver to assess inferior glenohumeral laxity.

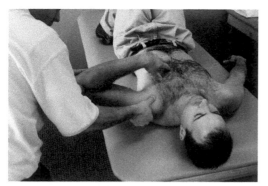

**Figure 2–4** Anterior drawer test.

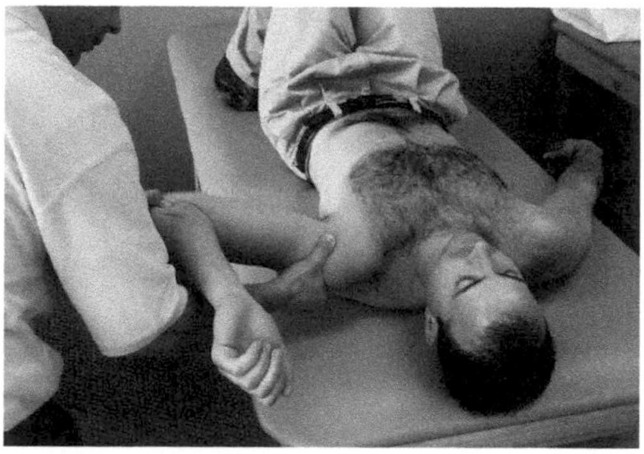

**Figure 2–5** Anterior fulcrum test.

with the patient positioned supine at the edge of the examination table and the arm abducted to 90 degrees. The arm is placed in maximal ER. In this position, the anterior band of the inferior glenohumeral ligament complex wraps around the anteroinferior aspect of the humeral head and acts as a hammock to prevent anterior humeral head displacement.[18] The examiner places the proximal hand on the posterior aspect of the glenohumeral joint to act as a fulcrum, while the other hand grasps the bicondylar axis of the elbow. The test is performed by simultaneously providing an anterior translation force as the humerus is brought into extension, acting as a fulcrum (**Fig. 2–5**). The examiner should feel minimal displacement and a firm end feel in the normal shoulder. In the patient with anterior micro-instability, there will be excessive anterior displacement and a softer end feel.

As discussed previously, overhead athletes with micro-instability often have internal impingement. Meister et al[15] originally described the internal impingement sign in which the patient is supine with the humerus at 90 degrees of abduction. The examiner passively rotates the shoulder into maximal ER until the patient experiences symptoms. Rather than feeling symptoms in the anterior aspect of the shoulder, which is common in patients with anterior macro-instability, the patient with internal impingement will have symptoms located specifically over the posterosuperior aspect of the shoulder. A relocation maneuver is then performed while the patient is in maximal ER. The examiner provides a posterior force to relocate the humeral head

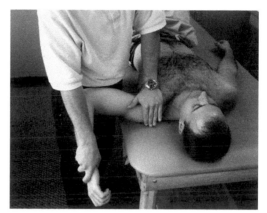

**Figure 2–6** Relocation maneuver performed during the internal impingement sign.

within the glenoid and effectively alleviate symptoms, signifying that the symptoms were related to anterior translation (**Fig. 2–6**).

### ◆ Rehabilitation Program for Overhead Athletes with Micro-Instability

The rehabilitation process for overhead athletes with micro-instability must restore ROM, muscular strength, and endurance as well as gradually restore proprioception, dynamic stability, and neuromuscular control. As the athlete advances, sport-specific drills are emphasized to prepare for a gradual return to competition through an interval sport program. Neuromuscular control drills are performed throughout; they are advanced as the athlete progresses to provide continuous challenges to the dynamic stabilizers and neuromuscular system. In the following section, we provide an overview of a functional rehabilitation progression for overhead athletes with microinstability, while incorporating the previously discussed principles and guidelines. The program is divided into four separate phases with specific goals and criteria to advance to the next phase. The use of a criteria-based rehabilitation program allows for the individualization of each patient and his or her specific pathology. It is imperative to modify each program based on the extent of each patient's pathology. Alterations in exercise activities, positioning, and rate of progression are based on the type of injury, healing constraints, and the tissues that are being stressed during rehabilitation.

## Acute Phase

The acute phase of rehabilitation begins either immediately following the injury or when symptoms arise. The duration of the acute phase is dependent on the healing constraints of the involved pathological tissues and the degree of the injury. The initial goals of the acute phase are to diminish pain and inflammation, normalize motion and muscular balance, and restore baseline proprioception and kinesthetic awareness.

One of the primary goals during the acute phase is to normalize total motion bilaterally. This often requires the addition of ROM and flexibility exercises for IR and ER in a restricted ROM based on the theory that motion assists in the enhancement and organization of collagen tissue, the stimulation of joint mechanoreceptors, and possibly the neuromodulation of pain. The rehabilitation program should allow for progressive applied loads, beginning with gentle passive ROM. Active-assisted range of motion (AAROM) exercises are performed by the patient, which include a cane or L-Bar (Breg Corp., Vista, CA) for flexion, ER, and IR. As the patient advances, flexion progresses as tolerated and shoulder rotation ROM is progressed from 0 degrees of abduction to 30, 45, and 90 degrees of abduction. In addition, pendulum, rope, and pulley exercises may be used as needed to facilitate additional motion.

We believe that one of the underlying causes of symptomatic internal impingement is excessive anterior shoulder laxity. One of the primary goals of the rehabilitation program is to enhance the athlete's dynamic stabilization abilities, thus, controlling anterior humeral head translation. In addition, another essential goal is to restore flexibility to the posterior rotator cuff muscles of the glenohumeral joint. We strongly suggest caution against aggressive stretching of the anterior and inferior glenohumeral structures. This may result in increased anterior humeral translation. As previously mentioned, the soft tissue of the posterior shoulder is subjected to extreme repetitive, eccentric contractions during the throwing motion. This may result in soft tissue adaptations and loss of IR ROM.[24] Common stretches performed include horizontal adduction stretching across the body with slight IR stretching at 90 degrees of shoulder abduction. The cross-body horizontal adduction stretch may be performed in a straight plane adduction motion as well as being integrated with a component of IR at the shoulder (**Fig. 2–7**).

Strengthening begins with submaximal, pain-free isometrics for shoulder flexion, extension, abduction, ER, IR, and elbow flexion. Isometrics are used to hinder muscular atrophy and restore voluntary muscular control while avoiding detrimental shoulder forces. Isometrics should be performed at multiple angles throughout the available ROM, with particular emphasis on contraction at the end of the currently available ROM.

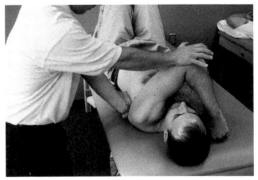

**Figure 2–7** Horizontal adduction stretch for the posterior cuff musculature.

Manual rhythmic stabilization drills are performed for the shoulder internal and external rotators with the arm in the scapular plane at 30 degrees and 45 degrees of abduction. Alternating isometric contractions facilitate co-contraction of the anterior and posterior rotator cuff musculature. Rhythmic stabilization drills may also be performed with the patient supine and the arm positioned at 100 degrees of flexion and 10 degrees of horizontal abduction. This position is chosen to initiate these drills because of the combined centralized line of pull of both the rotator cuff and the deltoid musculature at this angle, causing a humeral head compressive force during muscle contraction. Thus, the position of the deltoid is aligned theoretically to assist the rotator cuff in compressing the humeral head within the center of the glenoid fossa and provide dynamic stability. The rehabilitation specialist employs alternating isometric contractions in the flexion, extension, horizontal abduction, and horizontal adduction planes of motion.

Active ROM activities are permitted when adequate muscular strength and balance have been achieved. The therapist initiates active motion in the acute phase with basic proprioceptive joint reproduction exercises. With the athlete's eyes closed, the rehabilitation specialist passively moves the upper extremity in the planes of flexion, ER and IR, pauses, and then returns the extremity to the starting position. The patient is then instructed to reposition the upper extremity to the previous location. The rehabilitation specialist may perform these joint repositioning activities in variable degrees throughout the available ROM. The specialist should also note the accuracy of the patient's self-repositoning in the exercise.

Closed kinetic chain exercises are also performed during the acute phase. The integration of closed kinetic chain (CKC) exercises, or axial compression exercises, is another important principle in the rehabilitation of the overhead athlete with micro-instability.[33] CKC exercises are used to stress the joint in a weight-bearing position, resulting in joint approximation. The goal of this is to stimulate articular receptors and facilitate co-contraction of the shoulder force couples, thus, incorporating a combination of eccentric and concentric contractions to provide joint stability.

The athlete performs the initial exercises below shoulder level such as weight-bearing on a table while standing. The athlete may perform weight shifts in the anterior/posterior and medial/lateral directions. Rhythmic stabilizations may also be performed during weight shifting. As the athlete progresses, he or she may do weight shifts on a medium-sized ball placed on the table. Weight-bearing exercises are progressed from the table to the quadruped position.

Ice, high-voltage stimulation, iontophoresis, ultrasound, and nonsteroidal antiinflammatory medications may also be employed during this phase to control pain and inflammation as needed. This will allow for the progression of exercises in the following phases.

## Intermediate Phase

The intermediate phase begins once the athlete has regained near-normal passive motion and sufficient balance of strength of the shoulder musculature. Baseline proprioception, kinesthesia, and dynamic stabilization are also needed before progressing because emphasis will now be placed on regaining these sensory modalities throughout the athlete's full ROM, particularly at end ROM. The goals of the intermediate phase are to enhance functional dynamic stability, reestablish neuromuscular control, restore muscular strength and balance, and maintain full ROM.

ROM exercises are continued and the athlete is encouraged to perform active-assisted ROM with a cane or L-bar to maintain motion. Joint mobility is continuously assessed and joint mobilizations and self-capsular stretches may be performed to prevent asymmetrical glenohumeral joint capsular tightness.

Strengthening exercises are advanced to include ER and IR with exercise tubing at 0 degrees of abduction and active ROM exercises against gravity. These exercises initially include standing scaption in ER (full can), standing abduction, side-lying ER, and prone rowing. As strength returns, the program may be advanced to a program that includes full upper-extremity strengthening with emphasis on posterior rotator cuff and scapular strengthening, such as the Thrower's Ten Program (**Fig. 2–8**). This program has been designed based on electromyographic studies to elicit activity of the muscles most needed to provide dynamic stability, particularly in the overhead athlete.[22,23]

The rehabilitation specialist initiates rhythmic stabilization exercises during the early part of the intermediate phase. Drills performed in the acute phase may be progressed to include stabilization at end ROM and with the patient's eyes closed. Proprioceptive neuromuscular facilitation (PNF) D2 patterns are performed in the athlete's available ROM and progressed to include full arcs of motion. Rhythmic stabilization drills may be incorporated at various degrees of elevation during the PNF patterns to promote dynamic stabilization.

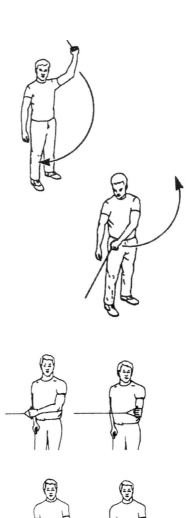

1A. **Diagonal Pattern D2 Extension:** Involved hand will grip tubing handle overhead and out to the side. Pull tubing down and across your body to the opposite side of leg. During the motion, lead with your thumb. Perform _____ sets of _____ repetitions _____ daily.

1B. **Diagonal Pattern D2 Flexion:** Gripping tubing handle in hand of involved arm, begin with arm out from side 45° and palm facing backward. After turning palm forward, proceed to flex elbow and bring arm up and over involved shoulder. Turn palm down and reverse to take arm to starting position. Exercise should be performed _____ sets of _____ repetitions _____ daily.

2A. **External Rotation at 0° Abduction:** Stand with involved elbow fixed at side, elbow at 90° and involved arm across front of body. Grip tubing handle while the other end of tubing is fixed. Pull out arm, keeping elbow at side. Return tubing slowly and controlled. Perform _____ sets of _____ repetitions _____ times daily.

2B. **Internal Rotation at 0° Abduction:** Standing with elbow at side fixed at 90° and shoulder rotated out. Grip tubing handle while other end of tubing is fixed. Pull arm across body keeping elbow at side. Return tubing slowly and controlled. Perform _____ sets of _____ repetitions _____ times daily.

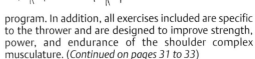
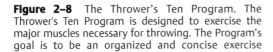

**Figure 2–8** The Thrower's Ten Program. The Thrower's Ten Program is designed to exercise the major muscles necessary for throwing. The Program's goal is to be an organized and concise exercise program. In addition, all exercises included are specific to the thrower and are designed to improve strength, power, and endurance of the shoulder complex musculature. (*Continued on pages 31 to 33*)

**2C. (Optional) External Rotation at 90° Abduction:** Stand with shoulder abducted 90°. Grip tubing handle while the other end is fixed straight ahead, slightly lower than the shoulder. Keeping shoulder abducted, rotate shoulder back keeping elbow at 90°. Return tubing and hand to start position.
I. Slow Speed Sets: (Slow and Controlled) Perform _____ sets of _____ repetitions _____ times daily.
II. Fast Speed Sets: Perform _____ sets of _____ repetitions _____ times daily.

**2D. (Optional) Internal Rotation at 90° Abduction:** Stand with shoulder abducted to 90°, externally rotated 90° and elbow bent to 90°. Keeping shoulder abducted, rotate shoulder forward, keeping elbow bent at 90°. Return tubing and hand to start position.
I. Slow Speed Sets: (Slow and Controlled) Perform _____ sets of _____ repetitions _____ times daily.
II. Fast Speed Sets: Perform _____ sets of _____ repetitions _____ times daily.

**3. Shoulder Abduction to 90°:** Stand with arm at side, elbow straight, and palm against side. Raise arm to the side, palm down, until arm reaches 90° (shoulder level). Perform _____ sets of _____ repetitions _____ times daily.

**4. Scaption, External Rotation:** Stand with elbow straight and thumb up. Raise arm to shoulder level at 30° angle in front of body. Do not go above shoulder height. Hold 2 seconds and lower slowly. Perform _____ sets of _____ repetitions _____ times daily.

**5. Side-lying External Rotation:** Lie on uninvolved side, with involved arm at side of body and elbow bent to 90°. Keeping the elbow of involved arm fixed to side, raise arm. Hold seconds and lower slowly. Perform _____ sets of _____ repetitions _____ times daily.

**6A. Prone Horizontal Abduction (Neutral):** Lie on table, face down, with involved arm hanging straight to the floor, and palm facing down. Raise arm out to the side, parallel to the floor. Hold 2 seconds and lower slowly. Perform _____ sets of _____ repetitions _____ times daily.

**6B. Prone Horizontal Abduction (Full ER, 100° ABD):** Lie on table face down, with involved arm hanging straight to the floor, and thumb rotated up (hitchhiker). Raise arm out to the side with arm slightly in front of shoulder, parallel to the floor. Hold 2 seconds and lower slowly. Perform _____ sets of _____ repetitions _____ times daily.

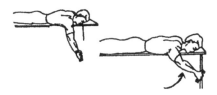

**6C. Prone Rowing:** Lying on your stomach with your involved arm hanging over the side of the table, dumbbell in hand and elbow straight. Slowly raise arm, bending elbow, and bring dumbbell as high as possible. Hold at the top for 2 seconds, then slowly lower. Perform _____ sets of _____ repetitions _____ times daily.

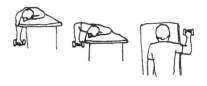

**6D. Prone Rowing into External Rotation:** Lying on your stomach with your involved arm hanging over the side of the table, dumbbell in hand and elbow straight. Slowly raise arm, bending elbow, up to the level of the table. Pause one second. Then rotate shoulder upward until dumbbell is even with the table, keeping elbow at 90°. Hold at the top for 2 seconds, then slowly lower taking 2 – 3 seconds. Perform _____ sets of _____ repetitions _____ times daily.

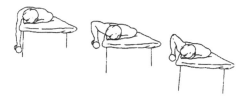

**7. Press-ups:** Seated on a chair or table, place both hands firmly on the sides of the chair or table, palm down and fingers pointed outward. Hands should be placed equal with shoulders. Slowly push downward through the hands to elevate your body. Hold the elevated position for 2 seconds and lower body slowly. Perform _____ sets of _____ repetitions _____ times daily.

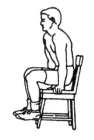

**8. Push-ups:** Start in the down position with arms in a comfortable position. Place hands no more than shoulder width apart. Push up as high as possible, rolling shoulders forward after elbows are straight. Start with a push-up into wall. Gradually progress to table top and eventually to floor as tolerable. Perform _____ sets of _____ repetitions _____ times daily.

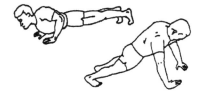

**Figure 2–8** (*Continued*) The Thrower's Ten Program. The Thrower's Ten Program is designed to exercise the major muscles necessary for throwing. The Program's goal is to be an organized and concise exercise program. In addition, all exercises included are specific to the thrower and are designed to improve strength, power, and endurance of the shoulder complex musculature.

9A. **Elbow Flexion:** Standing with arm against side and palm facing inward, bend elbow upward turning palm up as you progress. Hold 2 seconds and lower slowly. Perform _____ sets of _____ repetitions _____ times daily.

9B. **Elbow Extension (Abduction):** Raise involved arm overhead. Provide support at elbow from uninvolved hand. Straighten arm overhead. Hold 2 seconds and lower slowly. Perform _____ sets of _____ repetitions _____ times daily.

10A. **Wrist Extension:** Supporting the forearm and with palm facing downward, raise weight in hand as far as possible. Hold 2 seconds and lower slowly. Perform _____ sets of _____ repetitions _____ times daily.

10B. **Wrist Flexion:** Supporting the forearm and with palm facing upward, lower a weight in hand as far as possible and then curl it up as high as possible. Hold for 2 seconds and lower slowly.

10C. **Supination:** Forearm supported on table with wrist in neutral position. Using a weight or hammer, roll wrist taking palm up. Hold for a 2 count and return to starting position. Perform _____ sets of _____ repetitions _____ times daily.

10D. **Pronation:** Forearm should be supported on a table with wrist in neutral position. Using a weight or hammer, roll wrist taking palm down. Hold for a 2 count and return to starting position. Perform _____ sets of _____ repetitions _____ times daily.

Also performed during the intermediate phase is manual resistance ER. By applying manual resistance to specific exercises, the rehabilitation specialist can vary the amount of resistance throughout the ROM and incorporate concentric and eccentric contractions, as well as rhythmic stabilization drills at end range (**Fig. 2–9**). The application of manual resistance assists in the reinforcement of proper resistance, form, and cadence based on the symptoms of each athlete. As the patient regains strength and neuromuscular control, external and internal with tubing may be performed at 90 degrees of abduction. All stabilization drills may be advanced by removing the patient's visual stimulus.

Scapular strengthening and neuromuscular control are also critical to regaining full dynamic stability of the glenohumeral joint. Several authors have reported that neuromuscular control of the glenohumeral joint may be negatively affected by joint instability. Allegrucci et al[1] compared kinesthesia in the dominant and nondominant shoulders of overhead athletes and found a significant decrease in kinesthesia sense in the dominant extremity. A decrease in neuromuscular control has also been associated with muscular fatigue. Carpenter et al[7] observed the ability to detect passive motion of shoulders positioned in 90 degrees of abduction and 90 degrees of ER. Results indicate a decrease in the detection of both IR and ER movement following an isokinetic fatigue protocol. Voight et al[27] examined joint angle replication following an isokinetic fatigue protocol. The authors reported a significant decrease in accuracy following muscle fatigue when comparing both active and passive joint reproduction. In addition, Myers et al[16] studied the effects of fatigue on active angle reproduction at both mid- and end range of IR and ER. The authors report that fatigue of the shoulder rotators resulted in decreased accuracy at mid- and end ROM.

Isotonic exercises for the scapulothoracic (ST) joint are performed as well as manual resistance prone rowing. Neuromuscular control drills and PNF patterns may be applied to the scapula. The biceps brachii and the ST musculature may also play a role in dynamic stabilization of the glenohumeral joint, although debate exists within the literature.[2,32,34] Pagnini et al[20] have noted that contraction of the biceps brachii has a significant effect on glenohumeral translation, whereas Wilk and Arrigo[32] have stated that the ST musculature serves to assist in active glenohumeral stabilization by providing a base of support and maintaining a constant length-tension relationship of the muscles about the shoulder. Therefore, strengthening of the biceps and ST musculature is crucial during the rehabilitation program.

Closed kinetic chain exercises are also advanced. Weight shifting on a ball is progressed to a push-up on a ball or unstable surface on a tabletop.

The rehabilitation specialist performs rhythmic stabilizations at the upper extremity as well as the uninvolved shoulder and trunk to incorporate a combination of upper extremity

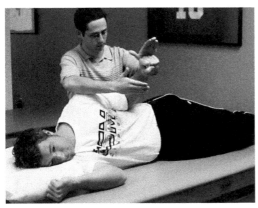

**Figure 2–9** Manual rhythmic stabilization drills performed during side-lying external rotation.

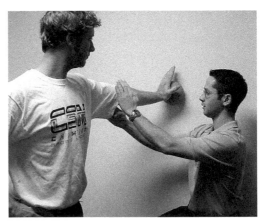

**Figure 2–10** Wall stabilization drills.

and trunk stabilization. Wall stabilization drills are performed with the athlete's hand on a small ball (**Fig. 2–10**). Further axial compression exercises include table and quadruped exercises using a towel around the hand, slide board, or unstable surface.

Lower extremity, core, and trunk strength are critical to perform overhead activities efficiently by transferring and dissipating forces in a coordinated fashion. Core stabilization drills are utilized to further enhance proximal stability with distal mobility of the upper extremity. Core stabilization is used based on the kinetic chain concept where imbalance within any point of the kinetic chain may result in pathology throughout. Movement patterns, such as throwing, require a precise interaction of the entire body kinetic chain to perform efficiently. An imbalance of strength, flexibility, endurance, or stability may result in fatigue, abnormal arthrokinematics, and subsequent compensation.

Therefore, the rehabilitation specialist also performs full lower-extremity strengthening and core stabilization activities during the intermediate phase. Basic exercises such as abdominal crunches and pelvic tilts are initiated during the late-acute phase to the early-intermediate phase. Exercises are progressed to include crunches with an altered center of gravity and with medicine ball throws.

In addition, the athlete may perform double- and single-leg balance on unstable surfaces such as foam or a balance beam. As core stability progresses, upper-extremity movement and medicine ball throws may be included to alter the athlete's center of gravity and train the athlete to control unexpected forces.

## Advanced Phase

The third phase of a functional rehabilitation program, the advanced phase, is designed to advance the athlete through a series of progressive strengthening and neuromuscular control activities while preparing the athlete to begin a gradual return to athletic activity. Criteria to enter this phase include minimal pain and tenderness, full ROM, symmetrical capsular mobility, good (at least 4/5 on manual muscle testing) strength and endurance of the upper extremity and ST musculature, and sufficient dynamic stabilization.

Full motion and capsular mobility are maintained through ROM and self-stretching techniques. These include manual stretching and L-bar exercises. Specific emphasis is placed on assuring that total motion remains equal bilaterally as the patient progresses throughout the rehabilitation program.

Strengthening exercises including the Thrower's Ten Program as well as exercises for the lower extremities and trunk are continued with a gradual increase in resistance. Exercises such as IR and ER with exercise tubing at 90 degrees of abduction may be progressed to incorporate eccentric and high-speed contractions.

The rehabilitation specialist may also initiate aggressive strengthening of the upper body depending on the needs of the individual patient. Common exercises include isotonic weight machine exercises such as bench press, seated row, and latissimus dorsi pull-downs within a restricted ROM. During bench press and seated row, the athlete is instructed not to extend the upper extremities beyond the plane of the body to minimize stress on the shoulder capsule. Latissimus pull-downs are performed in front of the head and the athlete is instructed to avoid full extension of the arms to minimize the amount of traction force applied to the upper extremities.

Plyometric activities for the upper extremity may be initiated during this phase as well to train the upper extremity to produce and dissipate forces. Plyometric exercises are used to provide a quick powerful movement involving a prestretch of the muscle, thereby activating the stretch-shortening cycle of the muscle.[35,37,38] Plyometrics replicate several functional movement patterns, such as throwing, that involve stretch-shortening cycles of the muscle tissue. The goal of which is to train the upper extremity to develop efficiently and withstand force, while simultaneously increasing neuromuscular control and core stability.

Stretch-shortening muscle contractions use a prestretching of the muscle spindles and Golgi tendon organs to produce a recoil action of the elastic tissues resulting in improved muscle performance by the combined effects of the stored elastic energy and the myotactic reflex activation of the muscle.

Plyometric exercises may provide several benefits to the overhead athlete, including increasing the speed of the myotactic stretch reflex, desensitizing the Golgi tendon organ, and increasing neuromuscular coordination. Furthermore, plyometrics serve as an excellent transitional exercise from slow isotonic movement to high-speed functional movements in throwing. Thus, the athlete will exhibit improved neural efficiency and coordination of muscle groups.

Initially, the athlete performs plyometric exercises using two hands. Specific exercises include a chest pass, overhead throw, and alternating side-to-side throw with a 3- to 5-pound medicine ball. Two-hand drills are progressed to one-hand drills as tolerated by the athlete, usually between 10 to 14 days following the initiation of two-hand drills. Specific one-hand plyometrics include baseball-style throws in the 90/90 position (90 degrees of abduction and 90 degrees of ER) with a 2-pound ball **(Fig. 2–11)** and stationary and semicircle wall dribbles. Wall dribbles are also beneficial to increase upper extremity endurance while overhead and may be progressed to include dribbles in the 90/90 position.

Axial compression exercises are progressed to include the quadruped and triped positions. Rhythmic stabilizations of the involved extremity as well as at the core and trunk may be applied. Unstable surfaces, such as tilt boards, foam, large exercise balls, or the Biodex stability system (Biodex Corp., Shirley, NY) may be incorporated to further challenge the athlete's stability system while in the closed chain position.

Dynamic stabilization and neuromuscular control drills are progressed to include reactive neuromuscular control drills and functional, sport-specific positions. Concentric and eccentric manual resistance may be applied as the athlete performs ER with exercise tubing with the arm at 0 degrees abduction. Rhythmic stabilizations may be included at end ROM to challenge the athlete to stabilize against the force of the tubing as well as the therapist. This exercise may be progressed to the 90/90 position to require the athlete to stabilize the shoulder at end range in a more sport-specific position **(Fig. 2–12).** In addition, rhythmic stabilizations may be applied at end range during the 90/90-position wall-dribble exercise. The athlete performs a predetermined number of repetitions before the therapist applies a series of rhythmic stabilizations at ER end ROM. These drills are designed to impart a sudden perturbation to the throwing shoulder at near end range to develop the athlete's ability to stabilize the shoulder dynamically to prevent the shoulder from translating into excessive ranges of motion.

Lower extremity and core strengthening and stability are continued. Exercises are progressed to provide further challenge and to include sport-specific positions. An unstable surface or balance beam may be used while performing upper extremity isotonic, manual resistance, and plyometric exercises to challenge core stability while performing upper extremity movements **(Fig. 2–13)**.

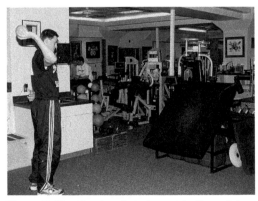

**Figure 2–11** One-handed plyometric throw into a trampoline using a 2-pound medicine ball.

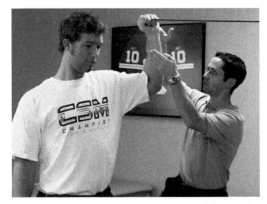

**Figure 2–12** Rhythmic stabilization drills in the 90/90 position (90 degrees of abduction and 90 degrees of external rotation) while the athlete performs resisted external rotation and internal rotation with exercise tubing.

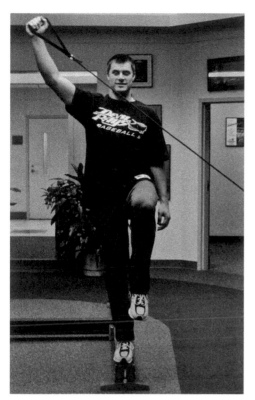

**Figure 2–13** Core strengthening and stabilization while the athlete performs resisted proprioceptive neuromuscular facilitation (PNF) D2 patterns on an unstable surface.

Near the end of the advanced phase, the athlete may begin basic sport-specific drills. Various activities such as underweight and overweight ball throwing or implement swinging for baseball and tennis players may be performed.

### Return to Activity Phase

Upon completion of the previously outlined rehabilitation program and the successful evaluation of the shoulder, the athlete may begin the final phase of the rehabilitation program, the return to activity phase. Specific criteria during the clinical exam that need to be fulfilled to begin an interval sport program include minimal complaints of pain or tenderness, full ROM, balanced capsular mobility, adequate proprioception, dynamic stabilization, and neuromuscular control, and full muscular strength and endurance based on an isokinetic examination. We routinely perform

a combination of isokinetic testing for our overhead athletes, which we refer to as the *Thrower's Series*.[30,31] Criteria to begin an interval sport program include an ER:IR strength ratio of 66 to 76% or higher at 180 deg/s, an ER to abduction ratio of 67 to 75% or higher at 180 deg/s.[30,31]

Interval sport programs are designed to gradually return motion, function, and confidence in the upper extremity after injury or surgery by slowly progressing through graduated sport-specific activities.[25] These programs are intended to gradually return the overhead athletes to full athletic competition as quickly and safely as possible. A detailed description of several interval sport programs can be found in chapter 9, "Use of Interval-Based Sport Return Programs for Shoulder Rehabilitation."

### ◆ Summary

Overhead throwing athletes typically present with a unique musculoskeletal profile. The overhead thrower frequently experiences shoulder pain due to anterior capsular micro-instability and increased demands placed on the dynamic stabilizers. This may be the result of repetitive high stresses imparted onto the shoulder joint and may lead to the development of injuries. Most commonly, these injuries are overuse injuries and can be successfully managed with a well-structured rehabilitation program. The rehabilitation program should focus on the correction of adaptive changes seen in the overhead thrower, such as loss of IR and muscular weakness of the external rotators and scapular muscles. The athlete may then initiate a gradual throwing program to return the thrower back to competition. Emphasis on enhancing proprioception, dynamic stability, and neuromuscular control is essential to achieve satisfactory outcomes in this particular group of patients.

### References

1. Allegrucci M, Whitney SL, Lephart SM, et al. Shoulder kinesthesia in healthy unilateral athletes participating in upper extremity sports. J Orthop Sports Phys Ther 1995;21:220–226
2. Andrews JR, Carson WG, McLeod WD. Glenoid labrum tears related to the long head of the biceps. Am J Sports Med 1985;13:337–341

3. Andrews JR, Timmerman LA, Wilk KE. Baseball. In: Pettrone FA, ed. Athletic Injuries of the Shoulder. New York, NY: McGraw Hill; 1995 pp. 323–341

4. Bigliani LU, Codd TP, Connor PM, et al. Shoulder motion and laxity in the professional baseball player. Am J Sports Med 1997;25:609–613

5. Brown LP, Niehues SL, Harrah A, et al. Upper extremity range of motion and isokinetic strength of the internal and external shoulder rotators in major league baseball players. Am J Sports Med 1988;16:577–585

6. Burkhart SS, Morgan CD, Kibler WB. Shoulder injuries in overhead athletes: the "dead arm" revisited. Clin Sports Med 2000;19:125–158

7. Carpenter JE, Blaiser RB, Pellizon GG. The effects of muscle fatigue on shoulder joint position sense. Am J Sports Med 1998;26:262–265

8. Crockett HC, Gross LB, Wilk KE, et al. Osseous adaptation and range of motion at the glenohumeral joint in professional baseball pitchers. Am J Sports Med 2002;30:20–26

9. Ellenbecker TS, Roetert EP, Bailie DS, et al. Glenohumeral joint total rotation range of motion in elite tennis players and baseball pitchers. Med Sci Sports Exerc 2002;34:2052–2056

10. Fleisig GS, Andrews JR, Dillman CJ, et al. Kinetics of baseball pitching with implications about injury mechanisms. Am J Sports Med 1995;23:233–239

11. Gerber L, Ganz R. Clinical assessment of instability of the shoulder. J Bone Joint Surg Br 1984;66:554

12. Harryman DT 2nd, Sidles JA, Harris SL, et al. Laxity of the normal glenohumeral joint: a quantitative in vivo assessment. J Bone Joint Surg 1992;1:113–118

13. Johnson L. Patterns of shoulder flexibility among college baseball players. J Athl Train 1992;27:44–49

14. Matsen FA, Harryman DT, Sidles JA. Mechanics of glenohumeral instability. Clin Sports Med 1991;10:783–788

15. Meister K, Buckley B, Batts J. The posterior impingement sign: diagnosis of rotator cuff and posterior labral tears secondary to internal impingement in overhand athletes. Am J Orthop 2004;33:412–415

16. Myers JB, Guskiewicz KM, Schneider RA, et al. Proprioception and neuromuscular control of the shoulder after muscle fatigue. J Athl Train 1999;34:362–367

17. Neer CS, Foster CR. Inferior capsular shift for involuntary and multidirectional instability of the shoulder. J Bone Joint Surg Am 1980;62:897–908

18. O'Brien SJ, Neves MC, Arnoczky SP, et al. The anatomy and histology of the inferior glenohumeral ligament complex of the shoulder. Am J Sports Med 1990;18:449–456

19. Osbahr DC, Cannon DL, Speer KP. Retroversion of the humerus in the throwing shoulder of college baseball pitchers. Am J Sports Med 2002;30:347–353

20. Pagnini MJ, Deng XH, Warren RF, et al. The effect of the long head of the biceps brachii on glenohumeral translation. Paper presented at: The Hospital for Special Surgery Fellows Research Symposium, August, 1993; New York, NY

21. Reagan KM, Meister K, Horodyski MB, et al. Humeral retroversion and its relationship to glenohumeral rotation in the shoulder of college baseball players. Am J Sports Med 2002;30:354–360

22. Reinold MM, Ellerbusch MT, Barrentine SW, et al. Electromyographic analysis of the supraspinatus and deltoid muscles during rehabilitation exercises [abstract]. J Orthop Sports Phys Ther 2002;32:A43

23. Reinold MM, Wilk KE, Fleisig GS 2nd, et al. Electromyographic analysis of the rotator cuff and deltoid musculature during common shoulder external rotation exercises. J Orthop Sports Phys Ther 2004;34:385–394

24. Reinold MM, Wilk KE, Reed J, et al. Change in shoulder and elbow range of motion of professional baseball pitchers before and after pitching. J Orthop Sports Phys Ther 2003;33

25. Reinold MM, Wilk KE, Reed J, et al. Interval sport programs: guidelines for baseball, tennis, and golf. J Orthop Sports Phys Ther 2002;32:293–298

26. Silliman JF, Hawkins RJ. Classification and physical diagnosis of instability of the shoulder. Clin Orthop Relat Res 1993;291:7–19

27. Voight ML, Hardin JA, Blackburn TA, et al. The effects of muscle fatigue on the relationship to arm dominance to shoulder proprioception. J Orthop Sports Phys Ther 1996;23:348–352

28. Walch G, Boileau P, Noel E, et al. Impingement of the deep surface of the supraspinatus tendon on the posterosuperior glenoid rim: an arthroscopic study. J Shoulder Elbow Surg 1992;1:238–245

29. Warner JJ, Deng XH, Warren RF, et al. Static capsuloligamentous restraints to superior-inferior translations of the glenohumeral joint. Am J Sports Med 1992;20:675–685

30. Wilk KE, Andrews JR, Arrigo CA, et al. The strength characteristics of internal and external rotator muscles in professional baseball pitchers. Am J Sports Med 1993;21:61–66

31. Wilk KE, Andrews JR, Arrigo CA. The abductor and adductor strength of professional baseball pitchers. Am J Sports Med 1995;23:307–311

32. Wilk KE, Arrigo C. Current concepts in the rehabilitation of the athletic shoulder. J Orthop Sports Phys Ther 1993;18:365–378

33. Wilk KE, Arrigo CA, Andrews JR. Closed and open kinetic chain exercises for the upper extremity. J Sport Rehabil 1996;5:88–102

34. Wilk KE, Arrigo CA, Andrews JR. Current concepts: the stabilizing structures of the glenohumeral joint. J Orthop Sports Phys Ther 1997;25:364–379

35. Wilk KE, Arrigo CA, Andrews JR. Functioning training for the overhead athlete. Sports Physical Therapy Home Study Course. LaCrosse, WI: Sports Physical Therapy Association; 1995

36. Wilk KE, Meister K, Andrews JR. Current concepts in the rehabilitation of the overhead throwing athlete. Am J Sports Med 2002;30:136–151

37. Wilk KE, Voight ML, Keirns MA, et al. Stretch-shortening drills for the upper extremities: theory and clinical application. J Orthop Sports Phys Ther 1993;17:225–239

38. Wilk KE. Conditioning and training techniques. In: Hawkins RJ, Misamore GW, eds. Shoulder Injuries in Athletes. New York, NY: Churchill Livingstone; 1996:333–364

39. Wilk KE, Meister K, Fleisig GS, et al. Biomechanics of the overhead throwing motion. Sports Med Arthrosc Rev 2000;8:124–134

# 3

# Rehabilitation of Macro-Instability

George J. Davies, Rob Manske, Robert Schulte, Christine E. DiLorenzo, Jason Jennings, and James W. Matheson

Neuromuscular dynamic stability of the shoulder is the key to functional performance. All joints in the body are dependent on stability being provided by static stabilizers (bones, ligamentous/capsular complex, labrum, noncontractile tissue) and dynamic stabilizers (the *muscular components* contractile unit of muscles and the proprioceptive/ kinesthetic system). When these systems work in harmony, the shoulder is one of the more marvelous joints in the body, particularly considering the demands placed upon it. The shoulder is expected to effectively place the hand in a position of function for a variety of tasks, including very delicate procedures such as performing surgery, powerful activities such as lifting hundreds of pounds overhead in Olympic weight-lifting, and sports-specific movements such as throwing a baseball over 90 mph with the shoulder exceeding 7000 to 9000 deg/s in angular velocity.[1] However, when there is an injury or dysfunction to any one of the aforementioned components, it disrupts the shoulder complex and creates impairments and functional limitations. Surgical interventions are usually required to correct osseous or ligamentous/capsular problems. Physical therapy interventions can significantly influence the remaining two components of shoulder stability, the muscular and proprioceptive systems, and often are very effective in treating patients with shoulder dysfunction. Coupling the components of the muscular and proprioceptive systems is what is described as *neuromuscular dynamic stability*.[2]

Instability of the shoulder is a common clinical entity that is encountered on a daily basis by the rehabilitation specialist. In this chapter, we discuss the unstable shoulder in relation to functional instability that occurs from noncontractile instability (which is the traditional approach) and functional instability that can occur from neuromuscular deficits, including musculotendinous weaknesses or proprioceptive/ kinesthetic deficits. We present the applications of motor-learning principles to rehabilitation, and explore the evidence-based approach to rehabilitation of the unstable shoulder. Additionally, several empirically based concepts that are regularly applied to shoulder instability rehabilitation will be discussed, including the contra-coup concept of shoulder instability, the posterior dominant shoulder, and a phased program with precise recommendations for focusing on neuromuscular dynamic stability. Several concepts and examples of motor-learning principles and how they can be applied to rehabilitation of the unstable shoulder are included.

Specifically, we present the concepts related to the examination, evaluation, diagnosis, prognosis, interventions, and treatment outcomes of the unstable shoulder. We also discuss the common mechanisms of injuries because the specifics of the injuries influence the nonsurgical as well as the surgical approaches to treatment, emergency care evaluation, treatment, and disposition. Additionally, we cover the traditional classifications of the unstable shoulder, which includes degree of instability, chronology of the instability, force required to create the instability, patient control over the instability, and direction of the instability. We also will briefly discuss various complications that can potentially influence the rehabilitation program, such as rotator cuff injuries, neurovascular triad injuries (including peripheral nerve injuries), Bankart lesions, bony Bankart fractures, and Hill–Sachs lesions. We present the evolution of immobilization of the unstable shoulder from duration and position in relation to its influence on the rehabilitation program. Recurrence rates and how they impact the rehabilitation process following the immobilization will be considered. In addition, we review the current literature emphasizing the 180-degree paradigm shift in how the anterior inferior instability should be immobilized and the anatomical and biomechanical rationale for the approach. We also present some visionary concepts of where we feel the future of rehabilitation for the unstable shoulder should be heading.

## ◆ Instability of the Shoulder

### Common Instabilities and Comorbidities

In the shoulder complex, particularly in relation to shoulder instabilities or common comorbidities, some terms and conditions include: traumatic, unilateral/unidirectional,

Bankart lesion, surgery (TU²BS); atraumatic, multidirectional, bilateral, rehabilitation, inferior capsular shift (AMBRI); acquired ligamentous/capsular laxity (ALL); superior labrum anterior posterior (SLAP) lesions; supraspinatus labral instability pattern (SLIP); glenohumeral internal rotation deficit (GIRD); scapula infera coracoid dyskinesia (SICK) scapula; anterior labral periosteal sleeve avulsion (ALPSA) lesions; partial articular supraspinatus tendon avulsion (PASTA) lesions; posterior labrocapsular periosteal sleeve avulsion (POLPSA) lesions; humeral avulsion of the glenohumeral ligament (HAGL) lesions; bony humeral avulsion of the glenohumeral ligament (BHAGL) lesions; superior labrum, anterior cuff (SLAC) lesions; avulsion of the anterior inferior glenohumeral ligament (AIGHL); glenoid rim articular divot (GARD) lesions; glenolabral articular disruption (GLAD) lesions; glenoid labrum ovid mass (GLOM) lesions, tensile undersurface fiber failure (TUFF) lesions; and traumatic humeral articular cartilage shear (THACS).

The presence of common comorbidities is particularly important to understand from the rehabilitation perspective. Often, the limiting factor in the rehabilitation program may not be the tissues involved from the primary instability problem, but in fact, from the tissue associated with the comorbidity, as in the case of a SLAP lesion.[3,4]

## The Mechanism of Injury

Several mechanisms of injuries compromise the integrity of the glenohumeral (GH) joint. The positions of the GH joint that usually result in an acute shoulder dislocation are (1) abduction/external rotation, (2) hyperflexion, (3) hyper-abduction, and (4) hyper-horizontal extension. The only way to identify the actual shoulder dislocation is when a radiograph documents the position of the humeral head relative to the surrounding anatomy. When the shoulder does dislocate, it is important to recognize that the majority of shoulder dislocations are actually intracapsular and create attenuation of the anterior inferior capsule.[5] This is one component of the Bankart lesion and has important implications to the postinjury immobilization position.

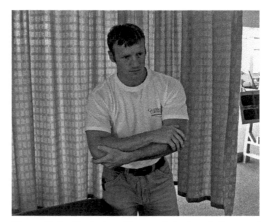

**Figure 3–1** Typical position and cluster of signs and symptoms of the patient after a traumatic anterior inferior dislocation.

## Patient's Clinical Signs and Symptoms

After an acute dislocation, the patient supports the arm away from the body and leans toward the side of the dislocation. There is an observable defect over the deltoid muscle area, often a palpable defect (humeral head) in the axillary area; there is pain from the pressure on the surrounding innervated structures (**Fig. 3–1**).

## Classifications of Shoulder Instabilities

Glenohumeral dislocations are classified according to the degree of instability, chronology, forces required to create the instability, patient's control, and the direction of the instability.

- *Degree of Instability*   The degree of instability or the instability continuum has several subclassifications ranging from the congenital laxity (multidirectional laxity), occult instability, micro-instabilities, multidirectional instabilities, subluxations, and luxations (dislocations).

- *Chronology of Instability*   The subcategories for the chronology include congenital, occult, acute, chronic/recurrent, and fixed/locked.

- *Force Required to Create the Instability*   Matsen et al[6,7] developed the original classification system used to describe the forces required to create the instability; the forces include TUBS and AMBRI. The first author of this chapter (GJD), however, recommends the TUBS acronym be modified to TU$^2$BS. As we have started to understand the shoulder better, we appreciate that the "U" should reflect both unilateral and *unidirectional*. To be consistent with the acronyms that describe the various types of instabilities, GJD coined the ALL acronym to represent an acquired ligamentous/capsular laxity, which are the adaptive changes that commonly occur in overhead athletes.

- *Patient Control over the Instability* The patient's control over the instability is predicated on whether the instability is voluntary or involuntary. The volitional shoulder instability is one where the patient can voluntarily subluxate and relocate his or her shoulder. The involuntary instability is when the patient does not have control over the instability and usually creates a functional instability.

- *Direction of the Instability* The only way to identify the actual shoulder dislocation is when a radiograph is taken and it documents the position of the humeral head relative to the surrounding anatomy. The directions of instabilities include the following: anterior (subglenoid, subcoracoid, subclavicular), inferior (inferior, anterior, posterior), posterior (subglenoid, subspinous, subacromial), superior, and multidirectional instabilities (MDIs). MDIs have more than one direction of instability associated with the condition.

## Complications of Shoulder Instabilities

- *Neurovascular Triad Injuries* Neurovascular triad injuries are common with anterior-inferior shoulder dislocations and often involve the axillary nerve. The patient occasionally ends up with an area of numbness on the lateral aspect of the shoulder.

- *Rotator Cuff Injuries* When the humeral head dislocates, it stresses the surrounding soft tissue structures and often creates partial or full thickness tears of the rotator cuff.

- *Bankart Lesions* Although there are various hybrids of the classic "essential Bankart lesion," it usually consists of a tearing of the labrum, attenuation of the anterior inferior capsule, and periosteal stripping of the subscapularis tendon from the neck of the glenoid fossa.

- *Hill–Sachs Lesions* A Hill–Sachs lesion is a contra-coup injury that results in an osteochondral compression defect of the posterior humeral head. A contra-coup injury means the injury actually occurs on the opposite side of where the obvious injury occurs. With the anterior dislocation, therefore, the Hill–Sachs lesion occurs on the opposite side, the posterior side of the joint on the posterior humeral head.

## ◆ Nonsurgical Treatment of Shoulder Instability

### Immobilization: Past and Present

In the past, immobilization of the GH joint was performed by using a sling or a swathe and sling with the arm in adduction (ADD) and internal rotation (IR). Traditionally, the duration of the immobilization times varied from a few days to 6 weeks. Recently, the trend has been to immobilize the shoulder until it is "ready"; "ready" is undefined.

Regardless of the amount of time the shoulder was immobilized, following a rehabilitation program, there was usually a high recurrence rate (30 to 90%). In most studies,[8–10] the recurrence rate was related to age: the younger the individual the higher the likelihood of redislocating the shoulder. This was because older individuals have decreased tissue mobility and consequently more limited motion, which makes them less vulnerable to reinjury. Furthermore, the lower redislocation rate in older individuals is also probably related to activity level and specific types of activities. Younger individuals are generally more active and more likely to participate in activities that will stress the joint more; whereas older individuals are less active and participate in activities less likely to place their arms in a compromising position where the arm is likely to redislocate.

Numerous shoulder braces are commercially available that try to stabilize the GH joint. This is one of the options available when treating

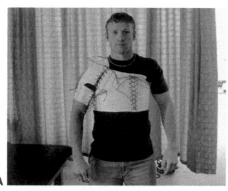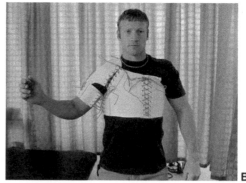

**Figure 3–2**  Denison-Duke Wyre Brace pictured **(A)** at rest and **(B)** with slight abduction and external rotation.

the unstable shoulder. There are limited scientific studies, however, that demonstrate that braces are effective in preventing redislocations. There are also few comparative studies demonstrating that one brace is better than another. In addition, taping and strapping techniques have been described in numerous athletic training books, manuals, and courses; but once again, there is limited scientific documentation to support any of the claims of the taping techniques. We have used numerous braces in our 30 years of clinical experience but have found the Dennison Duke-Wyre Shoulder Brace ([Brace International, Atlanta, GA] **Fig. 3–2**) to be the most effective for those athletes who wear the brace for a season, or who are injured during the season and want to finish the season before undergoing the elective surgery. For a complete discussion of shoulder bracing and taping methods, the reader is referred to chapter 8, "Use of Taping and External Devices in Shoulder Rehabilitation" for more detail.

The standard of care when someone dislocates the shoulder is to immobilize in adduction and internal rotation (ADD/IR), rehabilitate the patient, and return the person back to activity. Often, the patient will redislocate a second, a third, or more times. Then, the issue of whether surgery should be performed is discussed with the patient. Marx et al[11] have demonstrated that a patient who dislocates the shoulder is 10 to 20 times more likely to develop glenohumeral arthrosis in that shoulder than in the normal shoulder. The term *dislocation arthropathy* describes this condition.

Drawing an analogy to a patient who ruptures the anterior cruciate ligament (ACL),

we do not immobilize, rehabilitate, and then return the person back to activity and allow reinjury of the knee several more times until a definitive surgical approach is performed. Part of the reason is to prevent additional damage to other surrounding structures within the knee. Yet, based on the Marx et al[11] study, a patient who dislocates a shoulder one time has a higher incidence of future degenerative changes. Consequently, not only does the patient have the potential to get future chondrosis in the articular surfaces, but the potential to injure other structures and create additional comorbidities also exists. Therefore, complete rehabilitation and referral for surgical correction of the instability is often needed to prevent reinjury and to prevent injury to other structures in the shoulder complex.

Although the focus of this chapter is on non-surgical rehabilitation, we would be remiss if we did not also acknowledge the landmark article published by Arciero et al.[12] In a prospective randomized controlled clinical trials study whereby patients who had initial anterior inferior shoulder dislocations were treated with rehabilitation or an arthroscopic Bankart reconstruction, the initial treatment of early surgical intervention demonstrated significant reductions of redislocations compared with the patients who were treated with non-surgical interventions (immobilization and rehabilitation).

Rowe[5] demonstrated the recurrence rate does not depend on how long the shoulder is immobilized or how securely it is immobilized. Hovelius et al[8] indicated the shoulder never redislocates in 52% of patients after an initial dislocation, and recurrent dislocations spontaneously cease in 20% of patients with recurrent dislocations. The optimum duration of immobilization, however, still needs to be determined.

Moreover, 71% of all recurrent dislocations occur within the first 2 years and 9% from years 2 to 5. Consequently, there have to be other variables that are important in the postinjury treatment and immobilization of patients with traumatic anterior inferior GH dislocations.

It is likely that the poor outcomes after shoulder dislocation with rehabilitation have occurred because the position of shoulder immobilization has been inappropriate.

Itoi et al[13] performed a cadaveric study to identify the apposition of the Bankart lesion. The study demonstrated that the external rotation position at the neutral position provided better coaptation of the Bankart lesion than did the position of the conventional position of ADD/IR.

In a follow-up study, Itoi et al[14] demonstrated by magnetic resonance imaging (MRI) that the detached soft tissue, known as a Bankart lesion, is better coapted to the bone with the arm in external rotation (ER) than in IR. When comparing the ADD/IR position to varying degrees of ER, the apposition of the Bankart lesion structures was very different. In the traditional position (ADD/IR), the Bankart lesion was not approximated at all and consequently compromised the ability of the structures to heal. Whereas, when the arm was placed in 30 degrees ER, there was much better apposition of the Bankart lesion. The less ER, the less contact of the respective structures occurred. There was good apposition at 0 (neutral position), but this significantly decreased the coaptation of the Bankart lesion structures when IR was used. The study's conclusion was that immobilization of the arm in ER better approximates the Bankart lesion to the glenoid neck than does the conventional position of IR.

Miller et al[15] followed up with a research study by placing an electronic force transducer between the respective Bankart tissue structures. They confirmed with a force transducer contact study what the original cadaveric, radiographic, and MRI studies demonstrated. The results illustrated the following:

- Measured contact force between the Bankart lesion and the glenoid
- 60 degrees IR: no contact force

- 0 degrees: contact force increased
- 45 degrees ER: maximum contact force (83.5 g)

With these three studies as a scientific anatomical and biomechanical basis, Itoi et al[16] completed a prospective randomized controlled clinical trials study. Forty patients participated and 20 were randomized into the IR position and 20 into the ER immobilization position. Initially, Itoi et al[16] immobilized the patients in 30 degrees of ER; however, this much ER was not well tolerated by patients. It is likely that the higher the contact force, the higher the healing rate. However, the less ER the arm was placed in, the more comfortable it was for the patient. Moreover, from a practical standpoint, having the arm externally rotated in 30 or 45 degrees would create an awkward position of the arm for activities of daily living (ADLs).

Additionally, Itoi et al[16] arbitrarily placed the arm in 10 degrees ER because the Miller et al[15] study also showed positive contact of the Bankart lesion via the force transducers. The patients who were positioned in IR were immobilized in the conventional sling and swathe. The patients positioned in ER were immobilized using a wire mesh splint covered with sponge. Because of the healing process with soft tissue, granulation tissue fills the gap and unites the soft tissue within 7 to 10 days and increases in tensile strength within 3 weeks. Therefore, Itoi et al[16] empirically immobilized both groups in the respective positions for 3 weeks.

The compliance rate for those who were immobilized in IR was 75%. Those immobilized in ER was 80%. The follow-up results at 15.5 months demonstrated the recurrence rate (i.e., redislocation) in all patients in the study for the group immobilized in IR was 30%, whereas those immobilized in ER was 0%. The individuals under 30 years old (who usually have a higher recurrence rate than older individuals) who were immobilized in IR had a recurrence rate of 45%. However, those under the age of 30 who were immobilized in ER had a recurrence rate of 0%. Interestingly, even after a surgical stabilization procedure, there is approximately a 5 to 10% recurrence rate by 1 year.[9,10]

The ultimate functional outcome is the patient's ability to return to the premorbid state, particularly with higher levels of activities like sports. The results demonstrated that those who were immobilized in IR had a return to their previous level of sporting activities of 58%, whereas those who were immobilized in ER had an 82% return to sporting activities.

The evidence has been universal regarding a high failure rate (defined by recurrent dislocations/subluxations). Consequently, it is time to do something differently: The results of the proper immobilization to create better apposition of the Bankart structures hold a lot of promise based on the scientific anatomical and biomechanical studies as well as a clinical outcome study. Continued research is validating the apposition of the Bankart lesion with the externally rotated humeral position as opposed or in comparison with the ADD/IR position traditionally used. Hart and Kelly[17] used arthroscopic visualization to confirm approximation of the Bankart lesion in patients following shoulder dislocation. Based on the plethora of evidence we presently use the UltraSling (Smith & Nephew DonJoy, Carlsbad, CA) to achieve the proper immobilization of the patient. This sling supports the patient's arm and places the healing tissues into the ER position to provide apposition for the healing structures (**Fig. 3–3**).

This 180-degree paradigm shift in how to immobilize the unstable shoulder is an example of evidence-based practice. Paradoxically, the evidence in the literature indicates that we should *not be* immobilizing the shoulder in the traditional position of ADD/IR. We expect that over the next several years with proper immobilization resulting in better tissue approximation for healing, the rehabilitation programs for nonsurgical treatments are going

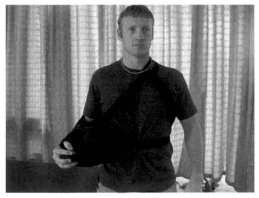

**Figure 3–3**   UltraSling.

to demonstrate significant improvements in outcome. The remainder of this chapter will focus on some of the causes of the shoulder instabilities, rehabilitation techniques, and guidelines to address these conditions.

## ◆ Causes of Shoulder Instability

Rehabilitation outcomes following shoulder instabilities will improve as we further understand some of the newer concepts of the causes of the occult and more-subtle instabilities. It is important that we identify the cause when we treat shoulder instabilities. Furthermore, it is important that we understand that with shoulder pathologies there often are several comorbidities. Moreover, as we better apply some of the concepts of motor learning principles to shoulder instability rehabilitation, we will see significant improvements in the outcomes.

How do we determine the cause of shoulder instability? Functional instability is the patient's inability to keep the humeral head centered in the glenoid fossa. The cause may be due to one problem or it may be multifactorial, consisting of noncontractile (bones, ligaments, capsule, and labrum) instability, contractile (muscles, tendons) weakness, or neuromuscular dynamic stability (proprioception/ kinesthesia) deficits. Each area needs to be tested with the particular deficits identified, and then each deficit needs to be addressed in the rehabilitation program.

### Noncontractile Instability

When considering shoulder stability provided by the static stabilizers, it is important to consider the shoulder as a circle concept. In other words, it is important to check both sides of the joint for any possible injuries that may contribute to the instability. This also introduces the *contra-coup concept* of shoulder injuries (in other words, the injury may also occur opposite to the side of the obvious injury). Although this chapter is primarily focused on macrotraumatic anterior inferior instabilities because they are the most common, it is also important to check the posterior capsular structures as well because they may also be injured.

The bones, ligaments, capsule, and labrum provide noncontractile stability. At the end of the range of motion (ROM), the ligaments and capsule are most active in providing stability because they are under tension. In mid-ROM, there is minimal tension and therefore the ligaments and the capsule do not play as significant a role in this position.

Ligament stability is dependent on position/specificity of ligament function and the capsular/ligamentous constraint mechanisms. Much of the capsular/ligamentous constraint mechanism is dependent on the position of the arm. When the arm is in the adducted position, the superior GH ligaments and superior capsule are taut. Whereas, when the arm is in the 90-degree abducted and 90-degree ER position, the anterior/inferior capsule and the inferior GH ligament are taut.[18]

## Examination of the Glenohumeral Joint for Instability

Joint laxity is *not* the same as instability. Joint laxity is the normal amount of translation of the joint for the individual patient. The patient has control over the joint; it does not subluxate/dislocate and is pain-free. In instability, the humeral head does subluxate/dislocate; the patient senses that and is apprehensive or has symptoms in the joint. We do not treat laxity; we treat instability.

The patient's history, subjective examination, mechanism of injury, epidemiological considerations, high index of suspicion, physical examination,[19–22] and imaging studies all contribute to the final diagnosis.[23] We primarily focus on a comprehensive physical examination of the shoulder[24,25] and use an algorithm-based examination for the special tests of the shoulder because it is clinically efficient.[27–29]

## Special Tests for Joint Instability

When performing this portion of the shoulder examination, the following examination criteria are evaluated:

- Degree of laxity/translation/instability
- Edge loading (this is the relationship of the head of the humerus to the edge of the glenoid fossa and is often used in grading laxity)[30,31]

- End feels (these are the sensations imparted to the hands of the examining clinician)
- Rebound compliance
- Crepitus/grating
- Locking/pseudolocking
- Clicking/clunking
- Reproduction of the patient's symptoms
- Apprehension

The degree of laxity is obviously unique to each patient. The best determination of normal, hypermobility, or hypomobility of the GH joint is to perform a bilateral comparison. However, there will occasionally be the patient who has had injuries to both sides. Then we need to rely on previous clinical experience and descriptive normative data. An example of early descriptive normative data for the GH load and shift test was published by Matsen et al[6] where they actually drilled percutaneous pins into the humerus and scapula and performed the testing under fluoroscopy to measure the amount of humeral head translation. They found the anterior load and shift produced $8 \pm 4$ mm; posterior load and shift $= 9 \pm 7$ mm; and the sulcus sign was $11 \pm 3$ mm.

Moreover, Borsa et al[32] studied the in vivo quantification of capsular end points in the nonimpaired GH joint using an instrumented measurement system. They found that it took $9.4 \pm .607$ pounds of pressure to hit the end point for the anterior load and shift test. The sulcus (inferior) test took $8.4 \pm 1.48$ pounds to reach the capsular end point. This study found that not much force is required when performing a physical examination of the shoulder.

The American Shoulder and Elbow Society's Classification[33] of shoulder laxity/instability is predicated on many of the previous concepts, such as edge loading and end feels (**Table 3–1**).

The physical examination of the shoulder using all the aforementioned concepts helps the clinician determine whether the ligamentous/capsular laxity or a labrum injury is contributing to the "instability." In the case of macro-traumatic injuries, as described in this chapter, ligamentous/capsular laxity or a labrum injury is often the patient's primary problem.

We primarily use the algorithm-based examination for the special tests of the shoulder as described by Davies et al[26] Schulte and Davies[28] and Ellenbecker[31] (**Figs. 3–4, 3–5**).

**Table 3–1** The American Shoulder and Elbow Society's Classification of Shoulder Laxity/Instability

| Grade | Glenohumeral Translation |
|---|---|
| Trace | Small amount of humeral head translation |
| I | Humeral head rides up the glenoid slope, but does not subluxate over the rim |
| II | Humeral head rides up and over the glenoid rim and dislocates, but spontaneously reduces when the stress is removed |
| III | Humeral head rides up and over the glenoid rim and dislocates, but remains dislocated on removal of the stress |

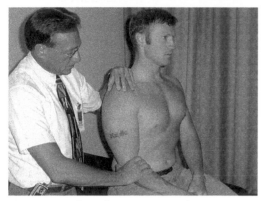

**Figure 3–4** Physical examination—sulcus sign at zero degrees.

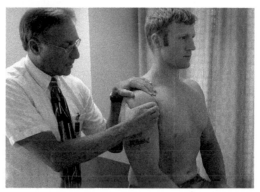

**Figure 3–5** Physical examination—anterior load and shift test.

## Contractile Stability: Muscle Strength, Power, and Endurance

Contractile stability is the functioning of the musculotendinous unit (MTU). Muscles provide more-dynamic stability at the middle of the ROM where the ligaments are lax. The MTU also provides stability at the end-ROM along with the ligaments/capsule due to the MTU tightening. As the MTU is lengthened, it provides a prestretch to the muscles based on the length:tension ratio and actually facilitates a muscle's ability to generate force.

The contractile stability, muscle strength, power, and endurance are commonly assessed with a variety of muscle performance testing, including manual muscle testing, hand-held dynamometry, cable tensiometers, isokinetic testing (**Fig. 3–6**), etc.[34–37]

Davies et al[34–37] and Ellenbecker and Davies[38] have published extensively on muscle performance, data analysis, and applications to clinical practice, particularly relative to the shoulder complex. Examples of data analysis include:

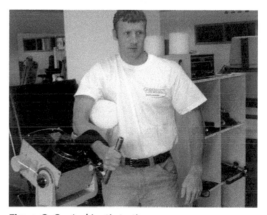

**Figure 3–6** Isokinetic testing.

- Specific measured parameters: peak torque, average power, total work, torque acceleration energy, etc.
- Bilateral comparison
- Unilateral ratio of agonist:antagonist
- Torque to body weight (relative/normalized data)

- Total arm strength (TAS), total body strength (TBS)
- Endurance analysis
- Normative data
- Functional correlation
- Sport-specific correlation

### Neuromuscular Dynamic Stability

Neuromuscular dynamic stability is the integrated functioning of the contractile stability along with the neurophysiological control system. This area focuses on the mechanoreceptors in the various structures, such as some of the sensors in the muscle–tendon units (muscle spindles, Golgi-tendon organs, etc.) and the sensors in the capsule and ligaments that control joint proprioception and kinesthesia (mechanoreceptors). Joint proprioception is reflective of joint-position sense, whereas kinesthesia is the control of joint movement. Neuromuscular dynamic stability is critical at all phases in the ROM due to the different receptors playing a role in the control of joint motion throughout the entire ROM.

#### Kinesthetic/Proprioception Testing

There have been several examples described in the literature as to how to test both proprioception and kinesthesia, including techniques using angular joint replication, end ROM reproduction, and threshold to sensation of movement.[39–45] Davies and Hoffman[39] have described joint angular replication testing in functional positions using minimal equipment so the testing can be performed in a busy clinical setting (**Fig. 3–7**).

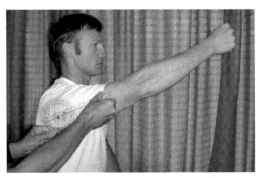

**Figure 3–7** Proprioceptive/kinesthetic testing.

### ◆ Kinesthetic Test Positions

**Table 3–2** Kinesthetic Testing Positions of the Shoulder

| |
| --- |
| Shoulder flexion <90-degree angle |
| Shoulder flexion >90-degree angle |
| Shoulder abduction <90-degree angle |
| Shoulder abduction >90-degree angle |
| Shoulder ER <45-degree angle |
| Shoulder ER >45-degree angle |
| Shoulder IR |

ER, external rotation; IR, internal rotation.

Smith and Brunolli[46] published the seminal article on joint proprioception and the effect of injuries on the receptors of the GH joint. Davies and Hoffman[39] followed with descriptive data measured on 100 normal males and 100 normal females: The composite normative data of seven test positions for the males and females was 3 degrees and 4 degrees, respectively. Lephart et al[41] in their Neer Award–winning article, documented the proprioceptive deficits in patients who had anterior instabilities in the shoulder. Following surgery and rehabilitation, they were able to demonstrate that the proprioceptive deficits were corrected and normalized to be comparable to the uninvolved side. Most of the research demonstrates that GH capsular/ligamentous injuries produce proprioceptive deficits to the shoulder.[41–43,47]

Davies et al,[48] Voight et al,[49] and Meyers et al[50] have demonstrated that muscular fatigue also has a detrimental effect on proprioception. They found that several factors can influence proprioception and consequently influence neuromuscular dynamic stability and functional performance. Therefore, proprioception must be assessed and, if deficient, strategies to address these deficits must be incorporated into the rehabilitation plan.

#### Closed Kinetic Chain Upper-Extremity Stability Test

As a result of these limitations in the literature for functional motor performance tests to check the shoulder complex, Goldbeck and Davies[51] have developed a shoulder stability series of tests, which includes the closed kinetic chain (CKC) upper-extremity (UE)

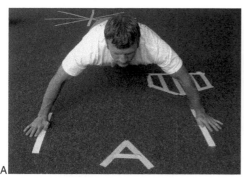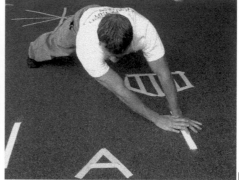

**Figure 3–8** **(A,B)** Closed kinetic chain upper-extremity stability test. **(A)** Start position, and **(B)** simulation of both hands on one line during the test.

stability test,[51] and the Functional Throwing Performance Index.[39] These tests are incorporated into a functional testing algorithm (FTA) of the shoulder complex.[52,53]

The specifics of the CKC-UE stability test (**Fig. 3–8**) are as follows. Two lines are drawn on the floor 3 feet apart. The patient performs a submaximal-to-maximal warm-up for ~15 seconds. Males perform the test in the push-up position, whereas females have the option of the push-up position or the modified position (from the knees). The patients then try to touch both hands to each line as many times as possible in 15 seconds. The patient performs three tests and the scores are averaged. The normative data developed over the past 10 years have demonstrated that males will touch an average of 21 times. Females, from the knee position, will touch an average of 23 times. Goldbeck and Davies[51] documented the reliability of the test by confirming intraclass correlation coefficients (ICCs) above 0.92.

### Functional Throwing Performance Index Test

Davies and Hoffman[39] developed the Functional Throwing Performance Index (FTPI) test, which is performed as follows (**Fig. 3–9**):

- Line on floor—15' from wall, 1' × 1' square, 4' from floor
- Four submax-to-max gradient controlled warm-up throws
- Controlled maximum number of accurate throws in 30 seconds

- Three sets are performed
- Divide total number/accurate number of throws × 100 = %
- Our descriptive normative data are described in **Table 3–3**.

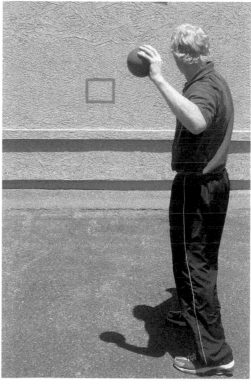

**Figure 3–9** Functional Throwing Performance Index (FTPI).

**Table 3–3** Descriptive/Normative Data for the Davies Functional Throwing Performance Index

|           | Males      | Females    |
|-----------|------------|------------|
| Throws    | 15         | 13         |
| Accuracy  | 7          | 4          |
| FTPI      | 47%        | 29%        |
| Range     | 33 to 60%  | 17 to 41%  |

FTPI, Functional Throwing Performance Index.

A reliability study demonstrated that the ICCs were above 0.90. Davies and Hofman[39] performed a test–retest reliability study with a 1-month interval of time between the tests. They found the ICCs to be all above 0.90. Furthermore, all the values fell within the described norms.

## ◆ Treatment of Shoulder Instability

### Ligamentous/Capsular Instability

If the primary cause of the functional instability is due to ligamentous/capsular laxity (noncontractile tissue that is injured), then the following types of treatment strategies are used: bracing, taping, muscle strengthening, proprioceptive/kinesthetic training, and neuromuscular dynamic stability.[54] If this is not successful in prevention of recurrent instability then surgery is often required.

### Musculotendinous Weakness

If the musculotendinous structures (contractile tissue) are injured and they create the functional instability, then the following types of treatment strategies are used: muscle strengthening, proprioceptive/kinesthetic training, and neuromuscular dynamic stability exercises. However, there is controversy in the literature demonstrating the success of treating patients with anterior inferior instabilities with therapeutic exercises alone. As previously pointed out, however, these patients were immobilized in the *incorrect positions of ADD/IR* and did not allow for coaptation of the injured Bankart tissue structures.

In a study by Burkhead and Rockwood,[55] 115 subjects were divided into five different cohorts: type I: traumatic subluxations—40 (34 anterior, 6 posterior), type II: traumatic with previous dislocation—34 (29 anterior, 5 posterior), type IIIA: voluntary subluxation with psychological problems—5 (3 anterior, 2 posterior), type IIIB: voluntary subluxation with no psychological problems—6 MDI (4 anterior, 2 posterior), type IV: involuntary subluxations—45 (33 MDI, 8 posterior, 4 anterior). The conclusions were that traumatic instability produced 15% good or excellent results (i.e., 85% redislocation or failure rate), whereas atraumatic subluxations had 83% good or excellent results.

In each subgroup, the patients who had posterior instability responded better than those who had anterior instability. These results are in contrast to other studies[56–60] that demonstrate posterior instabilities do not do as well with rehabilitation as do anterior instabilities.

In contrast, Von Eisenhart-Rothe et al[60] demonstrated that this muscle activity led to significant recentering in traumatic but not in atraumatic instability. The study also showed that in traumatic instability, increased translation was observed only in functionally important arm positions, whereas intact active stabilizers demonstrate sufficient recentering. In atraumatic instability, a decentralized head position was also recorded during muscle activity, suggesting alterations of the active stabilizers.

### Exercises for Rehabilitation of the Shoulder Complex

For the core strengthening exercises of the shoulder complex, the dynamic stabilization exercises that we incorporate include the Moseley et al,[61] exercises for the scapulothoracic (ST) area, the Townsend et al,[62] exercises for the GH area, Davies et al[39] rotator cuff exercises in the 30/30/30 (30 degrees of abduction, 30 degrees of scaption, and 30 degrees of a diagonal tilt) position, and the Davies and Ellenbecker[63] for TAS.

#### Scapulothoracic Exercises

The Moseley et al[61] exercises identified the four core exercises for the ST muscles, which included scaption with the thumb up for the

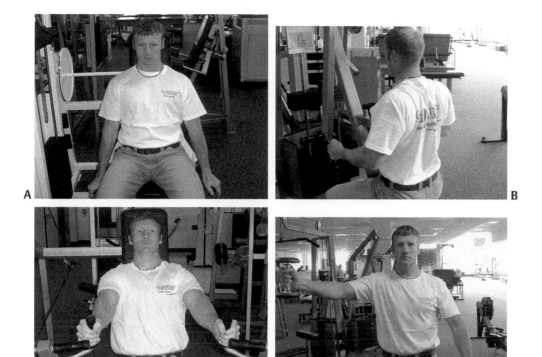

**Figure 3–10**    Four Moseley exercises in super-set format: **(A)** scapular depression, **(B)** seated row, **(C)** scapular protraction, and **(D)** scaption.

upper trapezius[64]; press-ups for the lower trapezius, latissimus dorsi, and teres major; push-up with a plus for the serratus anterior[65]; and scapular retraction for the middle trapezius and rhomboids. However, many different exercises can be used for strengthening the ST muscles[66–69] (**Fig. 3–10**).

### Glenohumeral Exercises

The Townsend et al[62] exercises identified the four core exercises for the GH muscles, which included scaption with the thumb down for the supraspinatus; press-ups for the lower trapezius, latissimus dorsi, and teres major; GH flexion for the anterior deltoid and the coracobrachialis; and external rotation with horizontal extension for the infraspinatus, teres minor, and posterior deltoid. However, in contrast to the scaption position with the thumb down, we recommend that the scaption position be performed with the thumb-up position based on the studies by Itoi et al[70] and

Takeda et al.[71] Itoi et al's[70] study demonstrated that the electromyogram (EMG) activity was similar in both the empty can (thumb down) and full can position (thumb up). More importantly, the thumb-up position was more comfortable for all subjects in the study. Takeda et al[71] used MRI scans to indicate that the thumb-up position was as effective as the thumb-down position for activating the supraspinatus (**Fig. 3–11**).

### Rotator Cuff Exercises (30/30/30 Position)

Davies and Hoffman[39] and Davies and Durall[72] originally described the concept of the 30/30/30 position for rotator cuff strengthening. As mentioned above, this position involved 30 degrees of abduction, 30 degrees of scaption, and 30 degrees of a diagonal tilt.[73]

The 30 degrees of abduction is used to protect the rotator cuff and prevent the wringing-out effect on the supraspinatus tendon.[74] If the arm is held in the adducted position, the

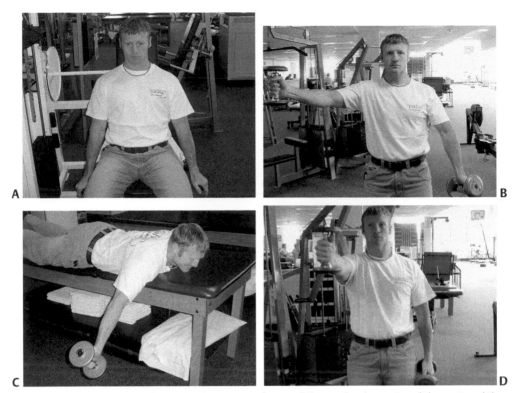

**Figure 3–11**   Four Townsend exercises in super-set format: **(A)** scapular depression, **(B)** scaption, **(C)** prone horizontal abduction with external rotation, and **(D)** shoulder flexion.

humeral head pushes on the articular side of the supraspinatus tendon creating a wringing-out effect on the tendon. If the arm is in the 90/90 (90 degrees of abduction and 90 degrees of external rotation) position, and the patient has weakness or pain inhibition of the force couple of the GH joint, has reflex inhibition of the rotator cuff muscles, or has a superior shear created by the deltoid muscle, then a wringing-out effect on the bursal side of the supraspinatus is caused by the coracoacromial ligament. The second 30-degree position places the arm into scaption because it is the functional position of the arm, protects the anterior inferior capsule, and prestretches the posterior rotator cuff muscles. By prestretching the posterior rotator cuff muscles (based on the length–tension curve), it facilitates their ability to generate power. The external rotator muscles are the weakest of the six directions of the GH joint. The 30-degree diagonal tilt prevents creating a posterior internal impingement

and is more comfortable for the patient than the transverse plane position when performing GH rotation exercises. Reinold et al[75] described the EMG activity of various exercises used to recruit the external rotator muscles. Graichen et al[76] performed an experimental in vivo study to test the potential changes of the subacromial space width during muscular contractions. Twelve healthy subjects were placed in an open MRI at 30, 60, 90, 120, 150 degrees of arm elevation. A force of 15 newtons caused an isometric contraction of the GH abductors or adductors. The results of the adducting muscle activity led to a statistically significant increase of the subacromial space width in all arm positions. These data show that the subacromial space can be effectively widened by adducting muscle activity and by affecting the position of the humerus relative to the glenoid. As a result, this effect may be employed for treatment of patients with an impingement syndrome.

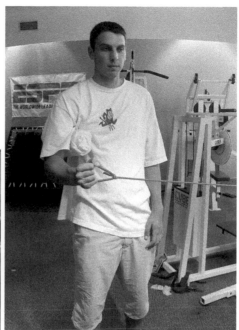

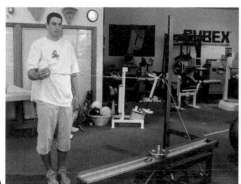

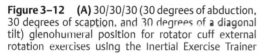

**Figure 3–12    (A)** 30/30/30 (30 degrees of abduction, 30 degrees of scaption, and 30 degrees of a diagonal tilt) glenohumeral position for rotator cuff external rotation exercises using the Inertial Exercise Trainer (Impulse Technology Newnan, GA), and **(B)** with elastic resistance. Note the use of a rolled towel to achieve this position and provide feedback for the patient.

In summary, the reasons to use the 30/30/30 position are:

1. It prevents the "wringing-out" effect.
2. The scaption position is a functional arc of motion for the shoulder.
3. The scaption position protects the anterior inferior capsule.
4. Scaption prestretches the ER (which are the weakest of the GH muscles) based on the physiologic length-tension curve.
5. It's a comfortable position for the patient to perform the IR/ER exercises.
6. Glenohumeral adduction to hold towel roll recruits EMG activity of the ER.
7. Glenohumeral adduction increases the width of the subacromial space.

A variety of exercises can be used to strengthen the rotator cuff. For example, Malanga et al,[77] Morrison et al,[78] and Sharkey and Marder[79] provide examples of exercises effective for isolating the rotator cuff and supraspinatus. We progress the patient to the 90/90 position to advance the rotator cuff strengthening program if the patient needs to use the arm in the overhead position[74,80–83] (**Fig. 3–12**).

### Total Arm Strengthening Exercises

Because the biceps brachii and triceps muscles cross the GH joint, they have the potential to contribute to dynamic stability of the GH joint. Davies and Ellenbecker[63] described a TAS effect of the entire upper-extremity musculature. Additionally, Pagnani et al[84] have shown how the biceps brachii functions to provide additional stability in the overhead athlete with underlying anterior GH joint instability (**Fig. 3–13**).

### Principles of Exercise and Their Application to Rehabilitation

#### Exercise Progression Continuum

Davies[34,35] described the exercise progression continuum as a means of integrative training and a safe and systematic process to

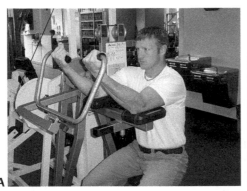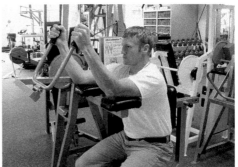

A                                                                                            B

**Figure 3–13**    Total arm strength (TAS) biceps. **(A)** Triceps, and **(B)** super-set format.

progress patients through an exercise progression program (**Table 3–4**).

## Muscle Balance through Super Sets

The balance of muscle activity functioning within the respective force couples of functional activity is often more important to produce normal functioning rather than isolated strength of individual muscles. As an example, Maggeray and Jones[85,86] demonstrated consistent activation of the rotator cuff prior to the more superficial deltopectoral muscles during isokinetic rotation in normal shoulders, confirming their role as dynamic stabilizers for the GH joint. Similarly, analysis of activation during rotation in the normal shoulder revealed that at least one component of the antagonist rotator cuff was always active providing evidence of their stabilizing role. Many activities actually involve the concepts of co-contraction to provide the appropriate joint stability.

Furthermore, an important part of normal function is the ability to dissociate different body parts during movement. Therefore, super sets are when the agonist muscle contracts during a set of reps followed by the antagonistic muscle. The advantages of using super sets are (1) it provides one muscle with a workout while the opposite muscle group undergoes relative rest, (2) it saves time because you do not have to have a recovery time for a muscle if performing several sets due to number 1, and (3) it works on muscle balance by exercising both agonist and antagonistic muscles.

## Cross-Education Training

With rehabilitation and training, increases in strength are not confined to the trained muscles but can even spread to the contralateral, untrained limb. As a generalization, the homologous muscles of the contralateral limb experiences a 10 to 15% increase in strength. Enoka[87,88] and Zhou[89] state that the strength gain in the contralateral limb is related to that achieved in the trained ipsilateral limb, with an average magnitude of ~60% of the ipsilateral strength gain.

## Bilateral Deficits

Studies by Henry and Smith[90] and Coyle et al[91] have found that when untrained subjects attempt such bilateral movements, the total force produced is less than the sum of the forces produced by the left and right limbs acting alone. This bilateral deficit is associated with a reduction in integrated electromyography (IEMG) in comparison to the same muscle active in the unilateral condition in agonists.

**Table 3–4**    Davies' Exercise Progression Continuum

Multiple-angle isometrics submaximal effort
Multiple-angle isometrics maximal effort
Short arc exercises submaximal effort
Short arc exercises maximal effort
Full ROM exercises submaximal effort
Full ROM exercises maximal effort

ROM, range of motion.

## Systematic Variable-Range Repetitions

Davies[34] described the concept of *progressive ranging* in 1984. Garfield[92] has expanded upon the concept and has developed the *RepMotions concept*, where a form of progressive ranging is performed but with several variations. When performing an exercise, Garfield has described the E2C (eccentric to concentric) impulse triangle.

At the end of the lowering of the weight, there is an extra force created to decelerate the weight, which is a deceleration impulse. To begin lifting the weight with each progressive increment in the ROM, extra concentric tension must be generated to provide enough force to overcome the inertia of the stationary weight that was just lowered. This extra force applied for a specified time is an acceleration impulse. When these deceleration and acceleration impulses are combined (E2C impulses), they help create more muscular tension. The greater the number of E2C switches during the exercise, the more times the E2C impulses are required, which results in increased muscle tension. By performing progressive ranging exercises, the intensity of the exercises is increased at each of the additional angles. Another variation of the progressive ROM (full ROM) is a variation called *step motion* (incremental partial ROM).[92]

## Progressive Range of Motion

By using partial ROM exercises to full ROM, it protects the soft tissue healing structures. Accordingly, the exercise ROM is gradually increased as the connective tissues progressively heal and can successfully accommodate greater exercise stress. Particularly in a patient with an unstable shoulder, training the eccentric/deceleration response is important to training the neuromuscular dynamic stabilization. It allows the patient to go progressively further into the compromised ROM in a controlled manner.[34,92]

Garfield[92] recommends advancing the RepMotions exercise program by varying the rules of intensity: the rule of spatial distribution and the rule of temporal distribution. The rule of spatial distribution indicates that the more joint angles that the E2C impulses are applied to, the more intense the exercise becomes. The rule of temporal distribution indicates the shorter the time between E2C impulses the more intense the exercise also becomes. There are numerous hybrids of the exercises that can be performed. By using exercises similar to these, a myoplasticity occurs; thus, morphological adaptations result in the muscle.

The neuromotor adaptations that occur include the following: increased IEMG, increased firing rate of motor units, increased recruitment of high-threshold motor unit and the time they can be activated, and increased motor unit coordination (neural facilitation, co-contraction of antagonists, synchronization of motor unit firing, and neural disinhibition).[93]

## Time Rate of Force Development/Force Development Quickness

This is a particularly important concept when developing neuromuscular dynamic stability to protect a patient with an unstable shoulder. One of the most important components of function is the ability to develop force rapidly. In many movements, a high rate of force development is a limiting factor to success. A related phenomenon is the so-called velocity specificity training. This facilitates rate coding and the onset of motor unit activation. Perhaps a neural adaptation to high-velocity training may consist of an acquired ability to increase the maximum motor unit firing rates in ballistic actions. Rhythmic stabilization/perturbation training may also help promote this ability in the muscles.

Irlenbusch and Gansen[94] performed muscle biopsies of the supraspinatus and deltoid muscle in patients who had involvement of the rotator cuff muscles. Their research demonstrated significant deficits occurring specifically to the fast twitch (FT) fibers of both the supraspinatus and deltoid muscles. Consequently, there are selective negative sequelae that occur to the FT fibers. Therefore, that raises the question as to how the FT fibers can be selectively recruited during the rehabilitation process. FT fibers can be preferentially recruited in two ways: (1) the all-or-none recruitment process with a maximum intensity effort, or (2) with fast movements. Sale[95,96] indicates that the larger FT motor units may be preferentially recruited over the smaller slow twitch units when rapid ballistic muscle actions are performed.

Davies and Hoffman,[39] over a decade ago, emphasized the importance of rhythmic stabilization exercises/perturbation training to enhance neuromuscular dynamic stability.

Consequently, Davies and Manske[97] and Manske and Davies[98] evaluated torque acceleration energy (TAE) in patients with shoulder dysfunctions. TAE is a measure of the explosive force created by muscular contractions and is important for the rapid force development and quickness that is required for functional activities. Following a rehabilitation program, using many of the concepts provided in this article, the results of this research demonstrated there was a significant improvement in most areas of TAE. Furthermore, most of the patients also normalized the involved side so it was within 10% bilateral comparison to the uninvolved side in TAE. This demonstrates that many patients with shoulder dysfunctions have TAE deficits that are amenable to change with appropriate interventions.

## What Is the Optimum Dosing for Therapeutic Exercise Programs?

Inevitably, the question arises regarding how much exercise is required. Several excellent references provide guidelines for the appropriate dosing of exercises:

1. Kraemer et al[99] provide the optimum resistance training guidelines and progression to be used in designing exercise programs for healthy adults.
2. Peterson et al[100] provide the optimum resistance training guidelines and progression to be used in designing exercise programs for athletes.
3. Wolfe et al[101] performed a meta-analysis of the literature comparing the single-set versus multiple-set resistance training programs. Their results demonstrate that single-set programs for an initial short training period in untrained individuals result in similar strength gains as multiple-set programs. However, as progression occurs and higher gains are desired, multiple-set programs are more effective. In contrast, trained individuals performing multiple sets generated significantly greater increases in strength than single sets.

4. Schroeder et al[102] compared 3 sets × 10 reps @ 125% intensity (MVC-1RM) versus 3 sets × 10 reps @ 75% intensity (MVC-1RM). Strength increases were 20 to 40% in both groups with no statistically significant differences. Consequently, submaximal eccentric training is optimal for musculoskeletal adaptations.
5. Pearson et al[103] present the National Strength and Conditioning Association's basic guidelines for the resistance training of athletes. Certainly one limitation is that most of these guidelines are based on healthy individuals rather than patients with various injuries, pathologies, or surgeries. However, without having particular guidelines on the injured population, we need to start with the best evidence available. The best evidence now is on normal populations, so we have to generalize until better information becomes available. See discussion above regarding the exercise progression continuum.

## Unique Concepts of Exercise and Their Application to Rehabilitation

### Contra-Coup Concept of Shoulder Stability (C3-S2)[23]

When rehabilitating most shoulder conditions, the external rotator muscles are harder to rehabilitate and get return of muscle power and function. Furthermore, if most clinicians were asked to select only one muscle to rehabilitate in a patient with a macrotraumatic anterior inferior instability, most would answer—the subscapularis—because it is the only anterior dynamic stabilizer of the GH joint.

However, if we were to use an analogy of a patient with an ACL insufficiency of the knee, rehabilitation would emphasize the hamstrings because they are synergistic with the ACL. This illustrates the contra-coup concept of dynamic stability. This is an example of the understanding of the shoulder being 10 years behind the knee.

Applying the contra-coup concept to the patient with an anterior inferior instability would be an example of dynamic stability. Cain et al[104] demonstrated the following results using electrical stimulation of the rotator cuff muscles and then evaluated the translation under fluoroscopy. The subscapularis contraction caused anterior translation of the humeral head, whereas the infraspinatus contraction caused posterior translation of the humeral head. Based on the above examples, the first author[39] (GJD) developed the contra-coup concept of shoulder stability to a posterior dominant shoulder to create dynamic stability The normal unilateral ratio of the GH IR:ER is a 3:2 ratio or 100%:66%. The normal unilateral ratio is modified to create the contra-coup concept of shoulder stability. Our operational definition of a posterior dominant shoulder is to increase the ER power by 10% thereby changing the ratio to 4:3 or 100%:76%.

Recently, Reinold et al[75] performed an EMG study to compare a variety of different exercises to selectively recruit the posterior muscles of the GH joint. Consequently, we use several of the examples described in that article to help develop the posterior dominant shoulder.[105] Of course, we do not achieve the ratio on all patients, but creating a posterior dominant shoulder is one of the most important goals to address the impairments, particularly in a patient with anterior inferior shoulder instability.

Additionally, the ROM and flexibility of the posterior shoulder need to be assessed, and if limited, then appropriate interventions used.[106]

# ◆ Neuromuscular Proprioceptive/Kinesthetic Deficits (Functional Neuromuscular Dynamic Stability)

In our opinion, this is where the future of shoulder functional neuromuscular dynamic reactive training really lies. Functional stability of the shoulder complex is dependent on neuromuscular dynamic control. The surrounding musculature and proprioceptive/kinesthetic systems must work in harmony to create a synergistic co-contraction to provide dynamic stability to the GH joint. Therefore, the challenge for clinicians is to implement motor-learning principles in a manner that enhances performance quality and learning in each rehabilitation phase. Motor-learning principles should promote the reacquisition of proper movement patterns by various methods and techniques. One of the difficult parts of rehabilitation is determining what structures needed for skill acquisition might have been damaged specifically to rehabilitate the involved structures. The clinician must first reactivate that feedback loop for lower level activities, such as postural support and ADLs before progressing to higher-level sport/work-related movement patterns. During the early phases of learning, there is a reorganization of the nervous system. The human nervous system must deal with the input of new information and instruction from the selected practice paradigm (rehabilitation program). The new information must be integrated into the central and peripheral nervous systems.

Trying to control an unstable shoulder dynamically with neuromuscular reactive training is predicated on facilitating the cybernetic system and producing muscle memory and motor engrams. Particularly when the arm is placed in a potentially compromising position, it is important that the muscles' engrams fire automatically quickly enough to control the movement. The pattern of movement, the force of propulsion, balancing by the stabilizing muscles, the duration of the propulsive phase, the relative positions of all the links of the body and the positioning of all links of the body after the movement are some of the many details that have to be preprogrammed into the brain. When sudden limb actions lasting less than ~0.2 seconds occur, feedback correction is invariably futile because reaction times are too long. Ballistic action requires the brain to estimate every detail of the movement in advance via feed-forward processes. Consequently, slow movements may be corrected readily by ongoing feedback information, but ballistic movements require the brain to determine every detail of the action in advance by mentally planning the exact sequence of neural activation for numerous individual muscles.

If the neuromuscular structures are injured, then the following types of treatment strategies are used in a four-stage approach to neuromuscular rehabilitation of the patient with anterior inferior instability.[107–110]

1. Proprioception and kinesthetic exercises
2. Dynamic (proactive) stabilization exercises
3. Reactive neuromuscular control
4. Functional skill movements and activities

## Stage 1: Proprioception and Kinesthetic Exercises (Baseline for Dynamic Stability)

The goals are to:

- Diminish pain and inflammation
- Normalize motion
- Restore proprioception and kinesthesia
- Establish muscular balance

The purpose of this stage is to create a baseline for dynamic stability. This is accomplished by first decreasing pain, inflammation, and swelling. Using nonsteroidal antiinflammatory drugs (NSAIDs) and various physical therapy modalities, such as interferential electrical stimulation, ultrasound, phonophoresis, iontophoresis, and cryotherapy can often be successful in decreasing pain, inflammation, and swelling. Then the focus of the rehabilitation is on restoring the normal joint arthrokinematics and normalizing the shoulder's physiological range of motion. If the noncontractile tissue is involved (capsule, ligaments, fascia, etc.), we recommend using the process described by Davies and Ellenbecker[111] where the total end-range time (TERT) formula facilitates an increase in the plastic deformation of the tissue. If the limitations are due to contractile limitations (muscle, muscle–tendon junction, tendon) then we recommend using static positional stretching, proprioceptive neuromuscular facilitation (PNF) contract-relax, or PNF hold-relax. After ROM is increased, particularly for the patient with the unstable shoulder, to have ROM available in the joint without the ability to provide dynamic control of the ROM is often dangerous and useless. The reason is that the patient has too much motion without dynamic control, which leads to recurrent instability of the shoulder joint. Consequently, after the ROM is normalized (or in the case of patients with instability such as described in this chapter), then utilizing proprioceptive and kinesthetic exercises to enhance dynamic stability along with muscle strength, power, and endurance exercises are utilized.

Basic proprioceptive exercises are used in the early stages of rehabilitation such as angular joint replications, threshold to sensation of movement, and end ROM reproductions. Submaximal, slow speed, pain-free rhythmic stabilizations (perturbations) in a nonprovocative position of the arm are implemented at this time. Proprioceptive feedback is extremely important for motor learning during all phases of rehabilitation.

Total body training and core stabilization exercises can also be implemented at this time along with scapular exercises, GH exercises, rotator cuff exercises, and TAS as outlined earlier in this chapter (Moseley et al,[61] Townsend et al,[62] Davies and Hoffman,[39] Davies and Ellenbecker[63]).

## Stage 2: Dynamic (Proactive) Stabilization Exercises

The goals are to:

- Maintain normalized motion and arthrokinematics
- Restore muscular balance
- Enhance dynamic functional stability
- Reestablish neuromuscular proactive control
- Rhythmic stabilizations (perturbations)

The clinical guidelines include[39]:
- Submaximal-to-maximal effort
- Slow to fast
- Known pattern

The primary purpose of this stage is to create *proactive* neuromuscular dynamic stability. The ROM is maintained and dynamic stability throughout the entire ROM is emphasized. The aforementioned exercises are continued using the super set concept to restore muscular balance to the shoulder complex. The proactive responses are exercises where the patient has control over the exercises that are being performed.

Examples would include exercises using the concept of rhythmic stabilizations (perturbations) with known patterns of resistance. Various clinical guidelines can be used to perform the rhythmic stabilizations, including a submaximal to maximal intensity effort exercise. Moreover, the speed of the exercises can vary from slow to fast movements. At this phase of the rehabilitation program,

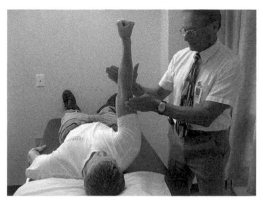

**Figure 3–14** Rhythmic stabilizations—open kinetic chain (OKC)—safe position.

the emphasis is on a known pattern so the patient has control over the exercises that are being performed (**Fig. 3–14**).

## Stage 3: Reactive Neuromuscular Control

The goals are to:

- Improve muscular power and endurance
- Enhance dynamic stability through proprioception and kinesthesia
- Improve reactive neuromuscular abilities
- Rhythmic stabilizations (perturbations)

The clinical guidelines include[39]:
- Submaximal to maximal effort
- Slow to fast
- Random patterns

- Advanced rhythmic stabilizations
- Eyes open to eyes closed
- Nonprovocative positions to provocative shoulder positions

Progressions from CKC—OKC (open kinetic chain) or OKC—CKC (**Fig. 3–15**)

- CKC exercises from stable to unstable surfaces (**Fig. 3–16**)
- CKC exercises from two arms to one arm

During this phase of the shoulder rehabilitation program, the emphasis switches to increase the power of the shoulder muscles, which builds on the strength base that was developed in the first two stages. Power is the ability to generate force quickly, which is more typical of many functional activities and almost all sporting activities. Proprioception and kinesthesia to create neuromotor stability are key components of this phase. Coupling the power with the kinesthetic training leads to improving neuromuscular reactive training and abilities.

Advanced rhythmic stabilization maneuvers performed at this time include visual feedback and no visual feedback. The patient's shoulder is usually progressed from a safe position to provocative positions where the shoulder is less stable and may often be placed into a compromising position. The patient can be progressed from OKC to CKC positions, or vice-versa, with the various advantages of each position capitalized on for the shoulder training. When in the CKC position, the patient

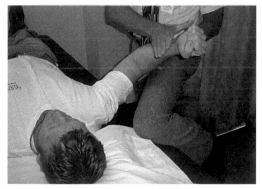

**Figure 3–15** Rhythmic stabilizations—open kinetic chain (OKC)—90/90 (90 degrees of abduction and 90 degrees of external rotation) position.

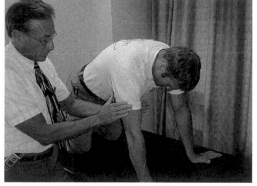

**Figure 3–16** Rhythmic stabilizations—closed Kinetic Chain (CKC) position.

is often progressed from a stable surface to an unstable surface using different equipment, such as tilt boards. The positions and stability of the patient can be modified (wall push-ups, kneeling push-ups, to push-up position) to progress the difficulty of the activity to incorporate the principles of progression and overload. Finally, the patient can progress from double-arm-support activities to single-arm-support activities.

### Stage 4: Functional Skill Movements and Activities

The goals are to:

- Maintain shoulder joint complex muscular balance
- Maintain reactive neuromuscular dynamic stability
- Gradual return back to activities, i.e., throwing

The primary focus at this stage of the rehabilitation program is to maintain the muscles' balance to provide the neuromuscular dynamic stability and to use a graduated progressive program for return to activity. This phase is where plyometric exercises are used

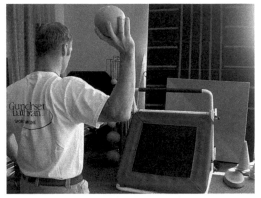

**Figure 3–18** Plyometrics—one arm—90/90 (90 degrees of abduction and 90 degrees of external rotation) position.

to replicate various functional activities. Research regarding the applications of plyometrics[112–114] and the applications of plyometrics to shoulder rehabilitation has been described.[115–117] The rehabilitation program is customized to meet the demands of the patient whether it's returning to ADLs, work, or sports (**Figs. 3–17, 3–18**).

### ◆ Summary

Treatment of the patient with GH joint instability requires a comprehensive evaluation and specific interventions aimed at ultimately restoring stability. A heavy focus on the dynamic stabilizers as well as neuromuscular control is needed to achieve this important goal. Recent research discussed in this chapter has provided guidance in the care and rehabilitation of patients with GH instability.

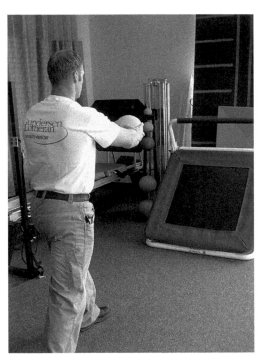

**Figure 3–17** Plyometrics—two arms.

### References

1. Pappas AM, Zawacki RM, Sullivan TJ. Biomechanics of baseball pitching: a preliminary report. Am J Sports Med 1985;13:216–222
2. Davies GJ, Kraushar D, Brinks K, Jennings J. Neuromuscular stability of the shoulder complex. In: Manske, R., ed. Rehabilitation for Post-Surgical Knee and Post-Surgical Shoulder Conditions. Amsterdam: Elsevier Science; 2006
3. Jennings J, Davies GJ, Tanner S, et al. Examination, surgery and rehabilitation of patients with superior labrum anterior and posterior (SLAP) lesions. In: Manske, R., ed. Rehabilitation for Post-Surgical Knee and Post-Surgical Shoulder Conditions. Amsterdam: Elsevier Science; 2006

4. Kim TK, Queale WS, Cosgarea AJ, et al. Clinical features of the different types of SLAP lesions. J Bone Joint Surg Am 2003;85-A:66–71

5. Rowe CR. Acute and recurrent dislocations of the shoulder. J Bone Joint Surg Am 1962;44-A:998–1008

6. Matsen FA 3rd, Harryman DT 2nd, Sidles JA. Mechanics of glenohumeral instability. Clin Sports Med 1991;10:783–788

7. Matsen FA, Lippitt SB, Sidles JA, Harryman DT. Practical evaluation and management of the shoulder. Philadelphia, PA: WB Saunders; 1994; pp. 59–110

8. Hovelius L, Augustini BG, Fredin H, et al. Primary anterior dislocation of the shoulder in young patients: a ten-year prospective study. J Bone Joint Surg Am 1996;78:1677–1684

9. Karlsson J, Magnusson L, Ejerhed L, et al. Comparison of open and closed arthroscopic stabilization for recurrent shoulder dislocation in patients with a Bankart lesion. Am J Sports Med 2001;29:538–542

10. Magnusson L, Kartus J, Ejerhed L, et al. Revisiting the open Bankart experience: a four- to nine-year follow-up. Am J Sports Med 2002;30:778–782

11. Marx RG, McCarty EC, Montemurno TD, Altchek DW, Craig EV, Warren RF. Development of arthrosis following dislocation of the shoulder: a case-control study. J Shoulder Elbow Surg 2002;11:1–5

12. Arciero RA, Wheeler JH, Ryan JB, McBride JT. Arthroscopic Bankart repair versus non-operative treatment for acute initial anterior shoulder dislocators. Am J Sports Med 1994;22:589–594

13. Itoi E, Hatakeyama Y, Urayama M, Pradhan RL, Kido T, Sato K. Position of immobilization after dislocation of the gleno-humeral joint: a cadaveric study. J Bone Joint Surg Am 1999;81:385–390

14. Itoi E, Sashi R, Minagawa H, Shimizu T, Wakabayashi I, Sato K. Position of immobilization after dislocation of the glenohumeral joint: a study with use of magnetic resonance imaging. J Bone Joint Surg Am 2001;83-A:661–667

15. Miller BS, Sannabend DH, Hatrick C, O'Leary S, Goldberg J, Harper W, Walsh WR. Should acute anterior dislocations of the shoulder be immobilized in external rotation? A cadaveric study. J Shoulder Elbow Surg 2004;13:589–592

16. Itoi E, Hatakeyama Y, Kido T, et al. A new method of immobilization after traumatic anterior dislocation of the shoulder: a preliminary study. J Shoulder Elbow Surg 2003;12:413–415

17. Hart WJ, Kelly CP. Arthroscopic observation of capsulolabral reduction after shoulder dislocation. J Shoulder Elbow Surg 2005;14:134–137

18. O'Brien S, Schwartz R, Warren R, et al. The anatomy and histology of the inferior glenohumeral ligament complex of the shoulder. Am J Sports Med 1990;18:449–456

19. Ellenbecker TS, Davies GJ. A comparison of three methods for measuring glenohumeral joint internal rotation. Sports Physical Therapy Section Newsletter. Fall 1999;4:13

20. Ellenbecker TS, Bailie DS, Roetert EP, Davies GJ. Glenohumeral joint total rotation range of motion in elite tennis players and professional baseball pitchers. Med Sci Sports Exerc 2002;34:2052–2056

21. Gould JA, Davies GJ, eds. Orthopaedic and Sports Physical Therapy. St. Louis, MO: CV Mosby; 1984

22. Sapaega AA, Kelley MJ. Strength testing of the shoulder. J Shoulder Elbow Surg 1994;3:3327–3345

23. Davies GJ, Ellenbecker TS. Focused exercise aids shoulder hypomobility. Biomechanics 1999;6:77–81

24. Davies GJ, Gould J, Larson R. Functional examination of the shoulder girdle. Phys Sportsmed 1981;9:82–104

25. Davies GJ, DeCarlo MS. Examination of the shoulder complex. In: Bandy WD, ed. Current Concepts in Rehabilitation of the Shoulder. Sports Physical Therapy Association Home Study Course. LaCrosse,WI: Sports Physical Therapy Association; 1995

26. Davies GJ, Wilk KE, Ellenbecker TS, et al. Study guide for the orthopaedic specialist examination. In: Examination and Treatment of the Shoulder: Orthopaedic Physical Therapy Section. Lacrosse, WI: Orthopaedic Physical Therapy Association. (In Press, 2006)

27. Davies GJ, Ellenbecker T, Heiderscheidt B, et al. Clinical examination of the shoulder complex. In: Tovin B, Greenfield B, eds. Evaluation and Treatment of the Shoulder: An Integration of the Guide to Physical Therapist Practice. Philadelphia: FA Davis; 2001; pp 75–131

28. Schulte RA, Davies GJ. Examination and management of shoulder pain in an adolescent pitcher. Phys Ther Case Reports. 2001;4:104–121

29. Matheson JW, Manske R, Davies GJ, eds. An Evidence-Based Algorithm Approach to the Examination and Treatment of Musculoskeletal Injuries. Amsterdam: Elsevier Science; 2006

30. Altchek DW, Warren RF, Wickiewicz TL, et al. Arthroscopic labral debridement: a three-year follow-up study. Am J Sports Med 1992;20:702–706

31. Ellenbecker TS. Clinical Examination of the Shoulder. Philadelphia, PA: Elsevier Saunders; 2004

32. Borsa PA, Sauers EL, Herling DE, et al. In vivo quantification of capsular end-point in the nonimpaired glenohumeral joint using as instrumented measurement device. J Orthop Sports Phys Ther 2001;31:419–431

33. Richards RR, An KN, Bigliani LU, et al. A standardized method for assessment of the shoulder. J Shoulder Elbow Surg 1994;3:347–352

34. Davies GJ. A Compendium of Isokinetics in Clinical Usage and Rehabilitation Techniques. Onalaska, WI: S & S Publishers; 1984

35. Davies GJ. A Compendium of Isokinetics in Clinical Usage and Rehabilitation Techniques. 4th ed. Onalaska, WI: S & S Publishers; 1992

36. Davies GJ, Ellenbecker TS. Eccentric isokinetics. Orthop Phys Ther Clin North Am. 1992;1:297–336

37. Davies GJ, Ellenbecker T. The scientific and clinical application of isokinetics in evaluation and treatment of the athlete. In: Andrews J, Harrelson GL, Wilk K, eds. Physical Rehabilitation of the Injured Athlete. 3rd ed. Philadelphia, PA: WB Saunders; 2004

38. Ellenbecker TS, Davies GJ. The application of isokinetics in testing and rehabilitation of the shoulder complex. J Athletic Training 2000;35:338–350

39. Davies GJ, Hoffman SD. Neuromuscular testing and rehabilitation of the shoulder complex. J Ortho Sports Phys Ther 1993;18:449–458

40. Hatterman D, Kernozek TW, Palmer-McLean K, Davies, GJ. Proprioception and its application to shoulder dysfunction. Critical Reviews Phys Rehabil Med. 2003;15:47–64

41. Lephart SM, Warner JJP, Borsa PA, et al. Proprioception of the shoulder joint in healthy, unstable, and surgically repaired shoulders. J Shoulder Elbow Surg 1994;3:371–380

42. Lephart SM, Pincivero DM, Giraldo JL, et al. The role of proprioception in the management and rehabilitation of athletic injuries. Am J Sports Med 1997;25:130–137

43. Lephart SM, Fu FH. Proprioception and Neuromuscular Control in Joint Stability. Champaign, IL: Human Kinetics Publishers; 2000

44. Myers JB, Lephart SM. The role of the sensorimotor system in the athletic shoulder. J Athletic Training. 2000;35:351–363

45. Pedersen J, Lonn J, Hellstrom F, et al. Localized muscle fatigue decreases the movement sense in the human shoulder. Med Sci Sports Exerc 1999;31:1047–1052

46. Smith RL, Brunolli J. Shoulder kinesthesia after anterior glenohumeral joint dislocation. Phys Ther 1989;69:106–112

47. Warner JJP, Lephart S, Fu FH. Role of proprioception in pathoetiology of shoulder instability. Clin Orthop Relat Res 1996;330:35–39

48. Davies GJ, Lawson K, Jones B. The acute effects of fatigue on shoulder rotator cuff internal/external rotation isokinetic power and kinesthesia [abstract]. Phys Ther 1993;73:S118

49. Voight ML, Hardin JA, Blackburn TA, et al. The effects of muscle fatigue on and the relationship of arm dominance to shoulder proprioception. J Orthop Sports Phys Ther 1996;23:348–352

50. Meyers JB, Guskiewicz KM, Schneider RA, et al. Proprioception and neuromuscular control of the shoulder after muscle fatigue. J Athletic Training. 1999;34:362–367

51. Goldbeck T, Davies GJ. Test–retest reliability of a closed kinetic chain upper extremity stability test: a clinical field test. J Sports Rehabil 2000;9:35–45

52. Ellenbecker TS, Manske R, Davies GJ. Closed kinetic chain testing techniques of the upper extremities. Orthopaedic Physical Therapy Clinics of North America 2000;9:219–230

53. Ellenbecker T, Davies, GJ. Closed kinetic chain exercise: a comprehensive guide to multiple joint exercise. Champaign, IL: Human Kinetics Publishers; 2001

54. Guanche C, Knatt T, Solomonow M, et al. The synergistic action of the capsule and the shoulder muscles. Am J Sports Med 1995;23:301–306

55. Burkhead WZ Jr, Rockwood CA Jr. Treatment of instability of the shoulder with an exercise program. J Bone Joint Surg Am 1992;74:890–896

56. Hawkins RJ, Schulte JP, Janda DH, et al. Translation of the glenohumeral joint with the patient under anesthesia. J Shoulder Elbow Surg 1996;5:286–292

57. Itoi E, et al. Dynamic anterior stabilization of the shoulder with arm in abduction. J Bone Joint Surg Br 1994;76-B:834–836

58. McMahon PJ, Jobe FW, Pink MM, Brault JR, Perry J. Comparative electromyographic analysis of shoulder muscles during planar motions: anterior glenohumeral instability versus normal. J Shoulder Elbow Surg 1996;5:118–123

59. Pagnani MJ, Warren RF. Stabilizers of the glenohumeral joint. J Shoulder Elbow Surg 1994;3:73–90

60. von Eisenhart-Rothe RM, Jager A, Englmeier KH, Vogl TJ, Graichen H. Relevance of arm position and muscle activity on three-dimensional GH translation in patients with traumatic and atraumatic shoulder instability. Am J Sports Med 2002;30:514–522

61. Moseley JB, Jobe FW, Pink M, et al. EMG analysis of the scapular muscles during a shoulder rehabilitation program. Am J Sports Med 1992;20:128–134

62. Townsend H, Jobe FW, Pink M, et al. Electromyographic analysis of the glenohumeral muscles during a baseball rehabilitation program. Am J Sports Med 1991;19:264–272

63. Davies GJ, Ellenbecker TS. Upper extremity. In: Timm K, ed. Total Arm Strength for Shoulder and Elbow Overuse Injuries. Sports Physical Therapy Association Home Study Course. LaCrosse,WI: Sports Physical Therapy Association; 1993

64. Durall C, Davies GJ, Kernozek TW, Gibson MH, Fater DCW, Straker JS. The reproducibility of assessing arm elevation in the scapular plane on the Cybex 340. Isokinet Exerc Sci 2000;8:7–11

65. Decker MJ, Hintermeister RA, Faber KJ, Hawkins RJ. Serratus anterior muscle activity during selected rehabilitation exercises. Am J Sports Med 1999;27:784–791

66. Kibler WB. Role of the scapula in the overhand throwing motion. Contemp Orthop 1991;22:525–532

67. Kibler WB. The role of the scapula in athletic shoulder function. Am J Sports Med 1998;26:325–337

68. Kibler WB. Shoulder rehabilitation; principles and practice. Med Sci Sports Exerc 1998;30:S40–S50

69. Kibler WB. Management of the scapula in glenohumeral instability. Tech Shoulder Elbow Surg. 2003;4:89–98

70. Itoi E, Kido T, Sano A, et al. Which is more useful the "full can test" or the "empty can test" in detecting the torn supraspinatus tendon? Am J Sports Med 1999;27:65–68

71. Takeda Y, Kashiwaguchi S, Endo K, et al. The most effective exercise for strengthening the supraspinatus muscle: evaluation by magnetic resonance imaging. Am J Sports Med 2002;30:374–381

72. Davies GJ, Durall C. Typical rotator cuff impingement syndrome: it's not always typical. PT Magazine 2000;8:58–71

73. Durall C, Davis GJ, Kernozek TW, Gibson MH, Fater DC, Straker JS. The effects of training the humeral rotator musculature on scapular plane humeral elevation. J Sport Rehab 2001;10:79–92

74. Quincy R, Davies GJ, et al. Isokinetic exercise: the effects of training specificity on shoulder torque [abstract]. J Athletic Train 2000;35:S-64

75. Reinold MM, Wilk KE, Fleisig GS, et al. Electromyographic analysis of the rotator cuff and deltoid musculature during common external rotation exercises. J Orthop Sports Phys Ther 2004;34:385–394

76. Graichen H, Hinterwimmer S, von Eisenhart-Rothe R, Vogl T, Englmeier KH, Eckstein F. Effect of abducting and adducting muscle activity on glenohumeral translation, scapular kinematics and subacromial space width in vivo. J Biomech 2005;38:755–760

77. Malanga GA, Jemp YN, Growney ES, An KN. EMG analysis of shoulder positioning in testing and strengthening the supraspinatus. Med Sci Sports Exerc 1996;28:661–664

78. Morrison DS, Frogameni AD, Woodworth P. Nonoperative treatment of subacromial impingement syndrome. J Bone Joint Surg Am 1997;79:732–737

79. Sharkey NA, Marder RA. The rotator cuff opposes superior translation of the humeral head. Am J Sports Med 1995;23:270–275

80. Ellenbecker TS, Davies GJ, Rowinski MJ. Concentric versus eccentric isokinetic strengthening of the rotator cuff-objective data versus functional test. Am J Sports Med 1988;16:64–69

81. Kollwelter K, Davies GJ, et al. Effects of impulse inertial training of the shoulder internal and external rotators of the shoulder [abstract]. J Ortho Sports Phys Ther 2000;30:A-39

82. Mont MA, Cohen DB, Campbell KR. Isokinetic concentric versus eccentric training of shoulder rotators with functional evaluation of performance enhancement in elite tennis players. Am J Sports Med 1994;22:513–517

83. Treiber FA, Lott J, Duncan J, et al. Effects of Theraband and light weight training on shoulder rotation torque and serve performance in college tennis players. Am J Sports Med 1998;26:510–515

84. Pagnani MJ, Deng XH, Warren RF, et al. Role of the long head of the biceps brachii in glenohumeral stability: a biomechanical study in cadavers. J Shoulder Elbow Surg 1996;5:255–262

85. Maggeray ME, Jones MA. Specific evaluation of the function of force couples relevant for stabilization of the glenohumeral joint. Man Ther 2003;8:247–253

86. Maggeray ME, Jones MA. Dynamic evaluation and early management of altered motor control around the shoulder complex. Man Ther 2003;8:195–206

87. Enoka R. Muscle strength and its development: new perspectives. Sports Med 1988;6:146–168

88. Enoka RM. Neural adaptations with chronic physical activity. J Biomech 1997;30:447–455

89. Zhou S. Chronic neural adaptations to unilateral exercise: mechanism of cross education. Exerc Sport Sci Rev 2000;28:177–184

90. Henry FM, Smith LE. Simultaneous vs separate bilateral muscular contractions in relation to neural overflow theory and neuromuscular specificity. Res Q 1961;32:42–46

91. Coyle EF, Feiring DC, Rotkis TC, et al. Specificity of power improvements through slow and fast isokinetic training. J Appl Physiol 1981;51:1437–1442

92. Garfield D. RepsMotions: The Science of Enhancing Progressive-Resistance Training. Naperville, IL: Motioneering; 2004

93. Yue G, Cole KJ. Strength increases from the motor program: comparison of training with maximum voluntary and imagined muscle contractions. J Neurophysiol 1992;67:1114–1123

94. Irlenbusch U, Gansen HK. Muscle biopsy investigations on neuromuscular insufficiency of the rotator cuff: a contribution to the functional impingement of the shoulder joint. J Shoulder Elbow Surg 2003;12:422–426

95. Sale DG. Neural adaptation to resistance training. Med Sci Sports Exerc 1988;20:S135–S145

96. Sale DG. Neural adaptation to strength training. In: Komi PV, ed. Strength and Power in Sport. Oxford: Blackwell Scientific Publications; 1992 pp. 249–265

97. Davies GJ, Manske RC. The importance of evaluating muscle power (torque acceleration energy) in patients with shoulder dysfunctions. Phys Ther 1999;79:S81

98. Manske RC, Davies GJ. Postrehabilitation outcomes of muscle power (torque acceleration energy) in patients with selected shoulder conditions. J Sport Rehab. 2003;12:181–198

99. Kraemer WJ, Adams K, Cafarelli E, et al. American College of Sports Medicine position stand: Progression models in resistance training for healthy adults. Med Sci Sports Exerc 2002;34:364–380

100. Peterson MD, Rhea MR, Alvar BA. Maximizing strength development in *athletes*: a meta-analysis to determine the dose-response relationship. J Strength Cond Res 2004;18:377–382

101. Wolfe BL, LeMura LM, Cole PJ. Quantitative analysis of single vs multiple-set programs in resistance training. J Strength Cond Res 2004;18:35–47

102. Schroeder ET, Hawkins SA, Jaque SV. Musculoskeletal adaptations to 16 weeks of eccentric progressive resistance training in young women. J Strength Cond Res 2004;18:227–235

103. Pearson A, et al. The National Strength and Conditioning Association's Basic Guidelines for the Resistance Training of Athletes. Strength & Cond 2000;22:14–27

104. Cain PR, Mutschler TA, Fu F, et al. Anterior stability of the gleno-humeral joint: a dynamic model. Am J Sports Med 1987;15:144–148

105. Davies GJ, et al. Computerized isokinetic testing of patients with rotator cuff (RTC) impingement syndromes demonstrates specific RTC external rotators power deficits. Phy Ther 1997;77:5106

106. Davies GJ, Wilk KE, Ellenbecker TS. Invited commentary on article: Tyler TF et al. Reliability and validity of a new method of measuring posterior shoulder tightness. JOSPT 1999;29:270–272

107. Davies GJ. The need for critical thinking in rehabilitation. J Sports Rehabil 1995;4:1–22

108. Davies GJ, et al. Application of the concepts of periodization to rehabilitation. In: Bandy WD, ed. Current Trends in Therapeutic Exercise for the Rehabilitation of the Athlete. Sports Physical Therapy Association Home Study Course. LaCrosse, WI: Sports Physical Therapy Association; 1997

109. Davies GJ, Zillmer DA. Functional progression of a patient through a rehabilitation program. Orthopaedic Physical Therapy Clinics of North America 2000;9:103–118

110. Wilk KE, Arrigo C. Current concepts in rehabilitation of the athletic shoulder. J Orthop Sports Phys Ther 1993;18:365–378

111. Davies GJ, Ellenbecker TS. Focused exercise aids shoulder hypomobility. Biomechanics 1999;6:77–81

112. Fortun CM, Davies GJ, et al. The effects of plyometric training on the internal rotators of the shoulder. Phys Ther 1998;78:S87

113. Guanche C, Knatt T, Solomonow M, et al. The synergistic action of the capsule and the shoulder muscles. Am J Sports Med 1995;23:301–306

114. Schulte-Edelmann JA, Davies GJ, Kernozek TW, Gerberding ED. The effects of plyometric training of the posterior shoulder and elbow. J Strength Cond Res 2005;19:129–134

115. Davies GJ, Matheson JW. Shoulder Plyometrics-plyometrics. Sports Med & Arthroscopy Review 2001;9:1–18

116. Davies GJ, Ellenbecker TS, Bridell D. Upper extremity plyometrics as a key to functional shoulder rehabilitation and performance enhancement. Biomechanics 2002;9:18–28

117. Siff MC. Plyometrics and the brain: the missing dimension. Fitness and Sports Rev Internat 1994;29:129–133

# 4

# Rehabilitation of Adhesive Capsulitis

Terry Malone and Charles Hazle

One of the most challenging and confounding treatment entities is that of the frozen shoulder (adhesive capsulitis). Significant advances have occurred in treatment approaches to many shoulder pathologies; however, very little has changed in the past 25 years for the patient afflicted with this problem. In this chapter, we outline a recommended sequence of care for these patients based on our clinical experience and available evidence of interventional efficacy.

Authors do not use the same definition for frozen shoulder; this may account for the difference of care and success presented related to this pathology. We recommend dividing these patients into idiopathic (primary) and trauma/immobilized (secondary) groupings. Idiopathic patients often do not present until they notice significant loss of motion, whereas the trauma-based subjects develop significant "stiffness" after immobilization. These two groups require very different approaches to management. Although not well received, education of the idiopathic patient is critical to reasonable expectations as to treatment efficacy and timeframes for interventional success. We will address each group with pathogenesis, treatment concepts, and evidence-based clinical outcomes after providing a history of this condition.

## ◆ Idiopathic or Primary Frozen Shoulder

The first defined reference to this pathology may be attributed to Duplay who in 1872 described "periarthrite scapulohumerale"—the onset of which was attributed to subacromial bursitis.[1] The condition was better defined and treatment described by Codman in 1934.[2] He stated that these patients exhibited a slow onset, pain-disrupted sleep, painful and significant restriction of elevation and external rotation yet had a normal radiographic picture. Interestingly, he noted that these patients recover, with even the most difficult cases responding in about 2 years.[2] Although many changes have occurred over the past 75 years, his observations are still relevant today.

In 1945, Neviaser[3] introduced the term *adhesive capsulitis* when he discovered dense thickening of the capsule, particularly in the axillary fold. He also believed that there were "intraarticular adhesions"; hence, his naming of the condition. DePalma[4] reported that this syndrome was caused by bicipital tenosynovitis. In 1975, Reeves defined frozen shoulder as patients presenting with restricted motion in all directions, spontaneous onset of pain, and no apparent causation.[5]

The natural history has often included the description of symptom resolution over time. It should be noted that Codman's early work[2] is cited for this concept but his definition of resolution was not of an asymptomatic state but rather that the patients did not have permanent damage or deformity and that they were not disabled through the development of arthritis. Shaffer et al[6] evaluated 62 patients with long-term follow-up to determine the expected outcome. Interestingly, they found that patients returned to function but approximately half did so with mild pain and/or stiffness. More than half of the patients demonstrated restriction of active motion, with the greatest restriction seen in external rotation. These authors then questioned the long-held belief of this condition being self-limiting because more than half of these patients do have persistent loss of motion, although the loss does not appear to significantly impact shoulder function. This is reinforced by the work of Griggs et al[7] who followed 75 patients with idiopathic adhesive capsulitis treated with a four-direction stretching program providing a mean follow-up of 22 months. They found significant positive outcomes with high patient satisfaction, but there existed retained differences in pain and motion when compared with the uninvolved shoulder.

The reason for these persistent changes may be related to the observations of Bunker.[8] He examined via arthroscopy 35 recalcitrant idiopathic frozen shoulder patients. The consistent finding (31 of 35) was one of abnormal villous fronding of the synovium arising from the subscapularis bursa; the other four patients were very longstanding and actually had dense scarring of these same areas of the synovium/capsule. After a second arthroscopy that followed manipulation in 13 of these patients, 12 patients demonstrated avulsion of the capsule in the infraglenoid region. These findings are consistent with Wiley,[9] who used arthroscopic evaluation of 37 patients with primary frozen shoulders demonstrating a granulation scarlike appearance in the same region as described by Bunker. Segmuller et al[10] likewise found proliferative synovial tissue beneath the biceps and encompassing the subscapular recess in 24 primary frozen shoulder patients. The common feature in all of these studies is the development of proliferative synovial tissue in the subscapular recess extending to the rotator interval, which may ultimately become scarlike; this explains the loss of capsular volume and resultant decrease in range of motion (ROM). It also may help explain the ultimate outcome of a return to function but with residual loss of motion because the scar tissues may lack normal capsular extensibility.

Numerous concomitant conditions may predispose one to idiopathic frozen shoulder. Bunker[8] presents a compelling case for these patients having "Dupuytren's like disease." He shows many relationships with the links of frozen shoulder patients to Dupuytren's (fibromatoses conditions) because they found more than half in his series presenting with both conditions. Many authors have described a link to diabetes, with the most accepted values being a 10 to 20% incidence of frozen shoulder in diabetics. There is an approximate doubling of this incidence in insulin-dependent patients. Patients are typically 40 to 60 years of age, and there is a higher frequency in women than men, with a 2 to 5% incidence in the general population.[11] Also, those who develop bilateral frozen shoulders are even more likely to have diabetes.[8,11] These findings indicate that some type of capsular fibroplasia is the causative agent of idiopathic primary frozen shoulder.

## ◆ Secondary Frozen Shoulder

This condition is often marked by an acute onset associated with trauma that is followed by immobilization (desired and designed via cast or other intervention) or unintentional as in the patient restricting use and movement volitionally, resulting in loss of motion. Harryman et al[12] reiterate this through their recommendation of the designation "post-traumatic stiff shoulder." They further state that this group can be subdivided into the

causative trauma: injury, disease, or surgery. Treatment concepts for these patients will vary significantly; prevention is the rule in secondary designated subjects, whereas it is often not possible to prevent development in primary idiopathic patients. It should be noted that clinicians may exacerbate its development in primary idiopathic patients if lengthy immobilization in response to pain is imposed. Importantly, the trauma-related secondary designated patients typically present with a specific direction of limitation rather than the more complete or global loss exhibited by the primary frozen shoulder.

## ◆ Treatment Concepts

We will address treatment concepts and provide the existing evidence of their efficacy specific to patient type (primary versus secondary). Unfortunately, although numerous treatments have been espoused, the evidence of efficacy is limited and further clouded by the previously mentioned level of recovery that is the rule rather than the exception: The primary designated patients regain function regardless of treatment if adequate time is provided— although still exhibiting measurable loss of motion and having some discomfort with use.

### Treatments of Primary Frozen Shoulder

*Algorithm of Care*

Idiopathic primary patients have a sequence of progression of symptoms; therefore, the process can be divided into stages marked by the predominant symptoms at particular times. We prefer to use a four-stage sequence: painful, freezing, frozen, and thawing. In the painful stage, the patient complains of pain with motion and use of the shoulder. This pain is exacerbated by active use and can be quite significant, particularly at the end ROM. In response to the pain, patients have a tendency to restrict use, particularly at end or extreme ROM, thus setting in place the initiation of loss of motion.

In the freezing stage, there is a progressive loss of motion. Patients lose significant amounts of external rotation (ER), elevation, and internal rotation (IR). They lose the motion actively and passively, with capsular shortening or restraint becoming obvious and having global restriction. The patient will exhibit pain at the end of the available ROM, which then facilitates a continued loss of motion. The frozen stage is a mature form of the freezing stage with a residual loss of motion but without significant pain at the end of the available range of movement. The patient can move and use the shoulder pain-free in the residual ROM. The patient is not experiencing additional loss of motion but rather is in transition to the next stage.

The final stage is thawing. Patients begin to see an increase in their ROM; during this stage, physical therapy interventions can be quite helpful in assisting the return of motion.

The great challenge is enabling patients to accept that these stages will occur sequentially and that they will regain their motion and function, but it requires months and years rather than weeks. This is not the information desired by a patient experiencing limited motion—particularly when pain is still a significant factor. An interesting observation has been that male patients often seem to recover more quickly than female patients do. We believe this is related to the time of presentation to the clinician. Women present when they lose the ability to reach clothing buttons or snaps behind their back (loss of IR), which is earlier in the progression. Men usually do not present until they are unable to get their wallet from their rear pocket; that is when they are closer to the thawing phase, later in the sequence or progression.

Treatment must be stage-specific and include significant patient education. Patients must understand that the expression, "no pain, no gain" is not appropriate for their condition. Each stage will be approached related to the predominant problems and expected tissue reactions to intervention. We will present some common overall themes and then present recommendations for treatment associated with each stage.

## Analgesics and Anti-inflammatories

Multiple authors have recommended the use of analgesics and antiinflammatories, with some level of success in alleviating the overall pain associated with shoulder pain.[11,12] Our experience supports the observation of Lee et al[13]; patients did better when these agents

were combined with gentle exercises. The use of intraarticular injection has been shown to have mixed results in published studies[8] and in our experience. No definitive recommendations can be made regarding their use; pain relief seems to be more obtainable than increased motion or function. Oral agents may be used throughout the treatment stages, particularly to assist with sleep disturbances.

## Distension of the Capsule

Some clinicians have attempted to increase the capsular volume through injecting fluid under pressure until the constrained capsule is distended and ruptures. In our experience this process has been of limited long-term success and must be done in later stages (frozen or thawing) to be successful.

## Stretching

Stretching must be very carefully applied during the painful and freezing stages. It has been our experience that gentle stretching within the pain-free ROM is quite useful in all stages; more aggressive or forceful end-ROM exercise, however, can only be used during the frozen and thawing stages. In most patients, several sets or a short series of motion exercises should be done throughout the day rather than attempting to do a lengthy single session. In our experience, a program of three to five repetitions in five or more short sets dispersed throughout the day is more efficacious and better tolerated by most patients, particularly during the first two stages. For patients who are awakened by shoulder pain, a gentle motion program performed within the pain-free ROM facilitates their return to sleep. We use low loads, or stretch intensities, and longer durations when treating patients clinically, but this is typically during the thawing stage to facilitate the greatest possible return of ROM.

## Heating Modalities

The isolated use of heating modalities is probably used less today than in the past. Heating modalities were used to modulate pain and thus promote increased shoulder movement by the patient. The use of these modalities today is as a precursor to stretching to attempt to increase tissue temperature and thus extensibility. If you are attempting to use moist heat, we advise that you be sure to place it in the axilla (use a cervical-sized heating pack) to reach the anterior inferior fold most effectively.

### Strengthening Exercises

Some clinicians recommend using strengthening activities within the available pain-free ROM. It is our recommendation that the patient be encouraged to use the arm as much as possible but that independent strengthening exercises are of limited value. They may have a greater role during the late-thawing stage as patients reengage in higher levels of function.

### Manipulation

Many authors have recommended the use of manipulation in the treatment of recalcitrant frozen shoulder patients.[11,12,14–16] The success of the treatment is dependent on patient selection and timing of intervention. Because of complications (fractures, tendon ruptures, etc.), manipulation under anesthesia is best applied only in the most severe cases and, importantly, only after the patient has reached the frozen stage. Early manipulation during the freezing stage results in a proliferative response and continued loss of motion; however, it is effective when performed in the frozen stage. Diabetic patients have an inconsistent response to manipulation. Most patients manipulated during the frozen stage do experience a significant increase in motion, with release typically of the inferior capsule. Harryman et al,[12] Roubal et al,[14] Placzek et al,[15] and Ekelund and Rydell[16] describe a number of appropriate manipulation techniques. Our recommended approach is translational with constant controlled loading; it is encouraging when we perceive a crepitant release with an immediate significant increase in motion. **Figure 4–1** illustrates a modified technique for small–amplitude oscillations at the end ER range.

### Arthroscopic or Open: Surgical Release

In recalcitrant cases, typically after failed manipulation, surgical release of the capsule may be necessary. Open procedures were used

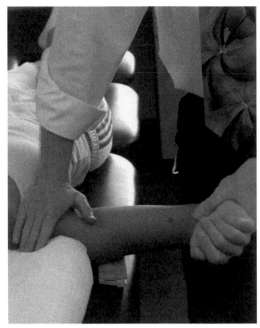

**Figure 4–1** Aggressive mobilization or manipulation of the glenohumeral joint must occur only after the frozen stage is present. This modified technique is tolerated relatively well. The therapist applies mobilization force through the scapula (pressure over the coracoid) at the end range of external rotation. The therapist receives feedback by watching the patient's face as controlled, small–amplitude oscillations are provided. Interestingly, the therapist can then follow these loads with physiologic stretches into external rotation through this position.

until the improvement in arthroscopic techniques; the majority of cases today are performed using the arthroscope. Harryman et al[17] and Warner et al[18] both demonstrated excellent outcomes via arthroscopic intervention in these difficult patients. For a detailed description of surgical intervention, refer to Harryman et al.[12]

### Treatment Recommendations and Efficacy

We recommend a stage-dependent approach to physical therapy management. Treatment concepts with special observations are shared with each patient. Our approach is an educational partnership with the patient, who must work with both a treating physician and a physical therapist in a joint commitment to treatment. Patients must be encouraged to stay "patient" with their treatment progress. Miller et al[19] and Diercks et al[20] both emphasize a similar approach in total management of these patients. In fact, the more aggressively treated patients exhibited less-positive outcomes than those who utilized supervised neglect.[20]

### ◆ Painful Stage

Often, patients do not present for treatment during this stage. They may attempt to link the pain to an activity or an abnormal sleeping posture. The true painful stage is when the patient does not use the arm for fear of pain. This stage may be quite short and, at times, it is not a significant event for the patient. Again, the patient often does not present during this stage.

If patients do present with pain, we recommend an approach of pain modulation (using a variety of techniques) and gentle ROM exercises performed in a few sessions daily. We have also used a "pillow on thorax" sleeping posture to provide relief. Pain modulation techniques include gentle distractions with perturbations and possibly the use of transcutaneous electrical neuromuscular stimulation (TENS) or other modulators to control pain. The ROM activities are typically what we call *the patient Codman*. Instead of asking the patient to relax in a flexed standing posture, we ask patients to grasp the involved arm's elbow with the uninvolved hand. They then raise the flexed arm forward supporting the weight of the arm with the uninvolved extremity. This seems to be tolerated more than the traditional Codman exercise by many patients.

For patients in significant pain, some physicians do provide an intraarticular injection with corticosteroid but this has limited impact on the treatment of the true primary frozen shoulder. It is vital that aggressive stretching or other active intervention not be attempted during this stage.

### ◆ Freezing Stage

During the freezing stage, the patient exhibits significant loss of motion (ER → elevation → IR). Patients have significant pain as they approach their end ROM and frequently decrease use of the arm to minimize pain. Treatment focus should be on maintenance of range while recognizing that a progressive loss of mobility is

the rule. Treatment should be gentle extension of the arm within the available range but not making the end range so painful as to elicit a significant painful response. Generally, we recommend three to five repetitions of movement done in five or more sessions daily. If patients are experiencing sleep disturbances, we recommend pillow on thorax positioning and gentle patient Codman if they are awakened by pain to facilitate return to sleep. Absolutely no aggressive stretching or resistive exercises should be performed during this stage. The patient must know that aggressive end-range exercise is counterproductive. Clinicians may educate the patient "to climb the wall" in the scapular plane as a gentle elevation-oriented ROM exercise. An interesting format for this activity is to place a strip of tape on the wall and floor to control and measure movement while minimizing the inherent substitution in this position.

### ◆ Frozen Stage

In the frozen stage, patients demonstrate a limitation of motion but experience relatively minimal pain. They can use their residual ROM and function within that range relatively well. If they wish to do strengthening, exercise done within the available range is often tolerated. It is our recommendation to continue their three to five sessions of daily "ranging" format to ensure that they do maintain their ROM and do not lose additional motion through lack of use. They can go to the end range more easily because there is much less pain or end-range sensitivity. If they have had a protracted process that has been ongoing for 6 or more months, in our experience manipulation can be done at this stage. It is vital that they do not have significant pain at end range (indicative of the freezing stage). You should ensure that they have reached the frozen stage before manipulation is performed; if not, a robust proliferative response ensues with a significantly negative outcome. We have also had less-positive responses in diabetic patients who have undergone manipulation, even in the frozen stage. Although there is less reaction at end range, we do not recommend attempting aggressive stretching but rather setting a regimen that will maintain their present ROM. If manipulation is performed, formal physical therapy visits are useful in maximizing the effect.

◆ **Thawing Stage**

The hallmark of the thawing stage is the return of motion. Interestingly, it is not the return of normal capsular volume because patients do not regain a normal capsule. They regain significant motion; some residual loss is present in about half the patients as described previously but this loss does not significantly limit functional activities. During this stage, physical therapists may use a variety of stretching maneuvers with success. We still prefer patients to do their three to five sessions daily but a limited number of physical therapy visits may be quite helpful in achieving their maximal return of motion. For treatment in this stage, we advise that you (1) mobilize the scapula—move the scapula over your fingers—don't dig your fingers under the scapula (**Fig. 4–2**); (2) mobilize the clavicle—bring your thumb horizontally into the posterior soft spot to move the clavicle anteriorly while the arm is supported (**Fig. 4–3**); and (3) use soft tissue techniques on the subscapularis, pectoralis minor, and external rotators to reduce their inherent muscle–tendon tension—you may use trigger point releases or deep tissue

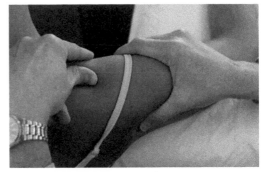

**Figure 4–3** Clavicular mobilization occurs in an anterior–inferior direction. The patient's arm must be supported, and the therapist applies the force with a horizontally aligned thumb. This is most helpful during the thawing phase, assisting in return of the last 30 degrees of elevation.

pressure approaches to minimize the restrictive nature of these structures prior to stretching patterns during the therapy sessions (**Figs. 4–4, 4–5**).

## Treatments of Secondary Frozen Shoulder

Treatment techniques for these patients are best provided through attempting to prevent their development. Early passive ROM within a protected range is paramount to avoiding these problems. When they are present, we address the specific direction of capsular

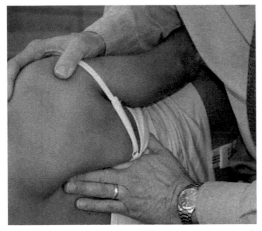

**Figure 4–2** Scapular mobilization is achieved with the arm in internal rotation, the arm supported, and the scapula moved over the fingers which are placed two finger widths above the inferior angle and medial to the medial border. The therapist moves the scapula over the fingers via lifting the shoulder as a unit. Gentle oscillations can also be provided. It is imperative that the fingers be above the inferior angle because the latissimus dorsi has an insertion into the inferior angle making an inferior approach uncomfortable. We often combine this process with pectoralis minor, external rotator, and subscapularis inhibitory techniques.

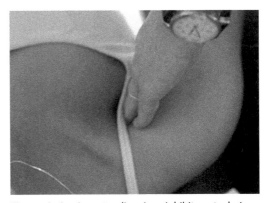

**Figure 4–4** A pectoralis minor inhibitory technique is performed through the therapist maintaining pressure to the underlying tendon as it approaches its coracoid insertion. We do not recommend the "strumming" techniques used by some clinicians. Typically, pressure is applied for 60 to 90 seconds until yielding is perceived.

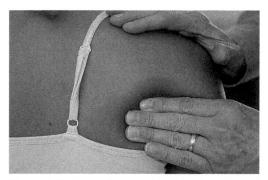

**Figure 4–5** External rotator inhibition is performed via a soft tissue vibratory pressure for 20 to 30 seconds. Passive internal rotation may be increased. This is often combined with a similar inhibition process to the subscapularis muscle.

restriction rather than the global approach required by the primary patients. For stretching portions of the capsule one should incorporate two factors: (1) Before applying load to the capsule—first decrease the resistance of the controlling muscle tendon units. Thus, if wishing to load (stretch) the posterior capsule, first manually vibrate over the external rotator muscle bellies for 20 seconds to reduce their muscle tone and allow loading to then be applied to the posterior capsule. (2) When wishing to stress capsule, add rotation to maximize loading—add IR to the posterior capsule stretch to increase its impact. You can use controlled stretching effectively with these patients, which is in direct contrast to primary frozen shoulder patients. Again, we recommend using specified routines of three to five repetitions repeated five or more times daily, but physical therapy sessions can be useful at this stage as well.

## ◆ Summary

This chapter provides detailed, evidence-based recommendations for the treatment of the patient with both primary and secondary frozen shoulder. Knowledge of the specific phases of this disease process, coupled with the combined efforts of the physician, physical therapist, and the patient, is required to enhance resolution of symptoms and provision of optimal care.

# References

1. Duplay S. De la peri-arthrites scapulo-humerale et des raideurs de l'epaule qui en sont la consequence. Arch Gen Med 1872;20:513
2. Codman EA. The Shoulder. 2nd ed. Boston: Thomas Todd; 1934
3. Neviaser J. Adhesive capsulitis of the shoulder: a study of pathological findings in periarthritis of the shoulder. J Bone Joint Surg 1945;27:211–212
4. DePalma AF. Loss of scapulohumeral motion. Ann Surg 1952;135:193–204
5. Reeves B. The natural history of the frozen shoulder syndrome. Scand J Rheumatol 1975;4:193–196
6. Shaffer B, Tibone JE, Kerlan RK. Frozen shoulder: a long term follow-up. J Bone Joint Surg Am 1992;74:738–746
7. Griggs SM, Ahn A, Green A. Idiopathic adhesive capsulitis: a prospective functional outcome study of nonoperative treatment. J Bone Joint Surg Am 2000;82-A:1398–1407
8. Bunker TD. Frozen shoulder: unraveling the enigma. Ann R Coll Surg Engl 1997;79:210–213
9. Wiley AM. Arthroscopic appearance of frozen shoulder. Arthroscopy 1991;7:138–143
10. Segmuller HE, Taylor DE, Hogan CS, Saies AD, Hayes MG. Arthroscopic treatment of adhesive capsulitis. J Shoulder Elbow Surg 1995;4:403–408
11. Malone TR, Richmond GW, Frick JL. Shoulder pathology. In: Kelley MJ, Clark WA, ed. Orthopedic Therapy of the Shoulder. Philadelphia: JB Lippincott; 1995
12. Harryman DT, Lazarus MD, Rozencwaig R. The Stiff Shoulder. In: Rockwood CA, Matsen FA, Wirth MA, Lippitt SB, eds. The Shoulder. 3rd ed. Philadelphia: Saunders; 2004
13. Lee M, Haq AM, Wright V, Longton E. Periarthritis of the shoulder: a controlled trial of physiotherapy. Physiotherapy 1973;59:312–315
14. Roubal PJ, Dobritt D, Placzek JD. Glenohumeral gliding manipulation following interscalene brachial plexus block in patients with adhesive capsulitis. J Orthop Sports Phys Ther 1996;24:66–77
15. Placzek JD, Roubal PJ, Freeman DC, Kulig K, Nasser S, Pagett BT. Long term effectiveness of translational manipulation for adhesive capsulitis. Clin Orthop Relat Res 1998;356:181–191
16. Ekelund AL, Rydell N. Combination treatment for adhesive capsulitis of the shoulder. Clin Orthop Relat Res 1992;282:105–109
17. Harryman DT II, Sidles JA, Matsen FA III. Arthroscopic management of refractory shoulder stiffness. Arthroscopy 1997;13:133–147
18. Warner JP, Allen A, Marks P, Wong P. Arthroscopic release for chronic, refractory adhesive capsulitis of the shoulder. J Bone Joint Surg Am 1996;78-A:1808–1816
19. Miller MD, Wirth MA, Rockwood CA. Thawing the frozen shoulder: the "patient" patient. Orthopedics 1996;19:849–853
20. Diercks RL, Stevens M. Gentle thawing of the frozen shoulder: a prospective study of supervised neglect versus intensive physical therapy in seventy-seven patients with frozen shoulder syndrome followed up for two years. J Shoulder Elbow Surg 2004;13:499–502

# 5

# Rehabilitation of Acromioclavicular Joint Injuries

Timothy F. Tyler and Michael J. Mullaney

Acromioclavicular (AC) separations usually occur because of a direct trauma to the superolateral region of the shoulder. The direct trauma is typically the result of an accident such as a skiing or biking mishap. Contact sports such as football, rugby, and hockey are also common causes of an AC separation. The superolateral aspect of the shoulder as it strikes the ground or is hit during a collision withstands a tremendous amount of stress. During this compression, the acromion is forced inferiorly, anteriorly, and medially, and transmits forces through the AC joint ligaments, thus possibly transferring stress to the coracoclavicular (CC) ligaments. In this chapter, we will discuss the anatomy, biomechanics, evaluation, and treatment of nonoperative AC injuries.

## ◆ Acromioclavicular Joint Anatomy and Biomechanics

The AC joint is a diarthrodial joint that joins the clavicle to the upper extremity via the scapula; it is a plane synovial joint with 3 degrees of freedom. The clavicle has ~50 degrees of rotation about its longitudinal axis, most of which is contributed by the mobile sternoclavicular (SC) joint.[1] The inclination of the joint can vary from vertical to 50 degrees of medial inclination with the clavicle overriding the acromion.[1] Although the clavicle rotates upward to 50 degrees during full overhead elevation (**Fig. 5–1**), only 5 to 8 degrees of the

motion is detected at the AC joint.[2] This difference is due to synchronous scapuloclavicular motion: As the clavicle rotates upward, the scapula rotates downward and the AC joint motion is minimized.[3] Interposed in the joint is a fibrocartilaginous disk that aids in distributing the forces from the upper extremity to the axial skeleton. Studies have shown that this disk has variable morphology in size, shape, and existence.[4]

The ligamentous complex and support of the AC joint stability is composed of intracapsular and extracapsular ligaments. The AC joint capsule is reinforced with an encompassing ligamentous complex (**Fig. 5–2**). Ligaments surround this joint on the anterior, posterior, superior, and inferior side. This complex acts as the primary restraint to posterior translation and axial distraction.[5] Fukuda et al[5] determined that during small displacements, the AC ligament complex is the primary restraint to posterior and superior displacements. As the displacement increases, however, the conoid ligament of the CC ligamentous complex becomes the primary stabilizer with superior clavicle translation, and the AC joint ligament complex remains the primary stabilizer to posterior translation (**Table 5–1**). The CC ligament consists of the lateral trapezoid ligament and the more-medial conoid ligament (**Fig. 5–2**). The fibers of this ligament travel from the inferior aspect of the clavicle to the base of the coracoid process and posteriorly to the pectoralis minor tendon attachment.[2] These two ligaments function differently with respect to

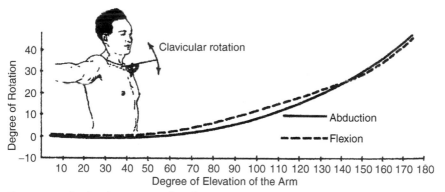

**Figure 5–1** The clavicle rotates to allow the arm to elevate overhead. (From Rockwood Jr, CA, Matsen F III. The Shoulder. Philadelphia, PA: WB Saunders; 1990: 213, Figure 6–7. Reprinted by permission. Figure originally from Inman VT, Saunders M, and Abbott LC. Observations on the function of the shoulder joint. J Bone Joint Surg 26, 1–30, 1944)

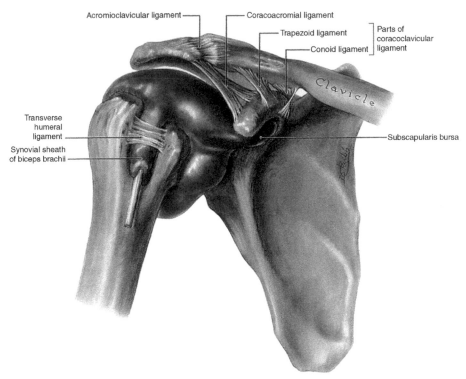

**Figure 5–2** Acromioclavicular (AC) joint stability is maintained by the AC ligament, coracoacromial ligament, and the two coracoclavicular ligaments. (From Agur AMR. Grant's Atlas of Anatomy. 9th ed. Baltimore, MD: Williams & Wilkins; 1991: 392, Figure 6.46. Reprinted by permission.)

**Table 5–1**  Primary Stabilizers of the Acromioclavicular Joint

| Direction of Force | Conoid Ligament | Trapezoid Ligament | AC Ligament |
|---|---|---|---|
| Anterior translation | Primary | | |
| Posterior translation | | | Primary |
| Superior translation | Primary | | |
| Distraction (axial) | | | Primary |
| Compression (axial) | | Primary | |

*Source:* From Lemos MJ. The evaluation and treatment of the injured acromioclavicular joint in athletes. Am J Sports Med 1998;26:137–144. Reprinted by permission. AC, acromioclavicular.

the direction of the loads applied. The conoid ligament functions as a restraint to anterior superior loading, whereas the trapezoid ligament functions as a restraint to posterior loading.[6] The CC ligament, though anatomically related to the AC joint and implicated in grade I and II AC joint separations, is the least important ligament to stability.[2] It primarily prevents anterosuperior translation of the humeral head when a rotator cuff pathology is present.[2]

## ◆ Classification of Acromioclavicular Joint Injuries

As discussed, each of the ligaments associated with the AC joint are responsible for maintaining a level of stability that promotes shoulder function. Each of the ligaments is responsible for maintaining joint stability in a specific

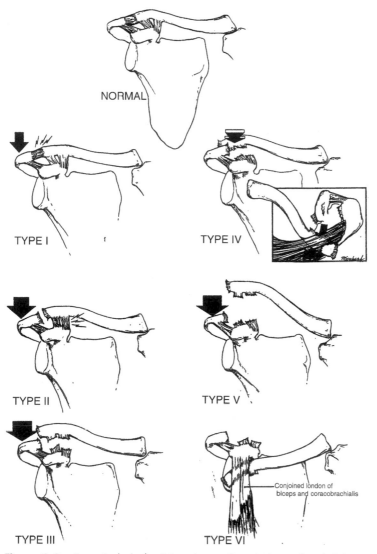

NORMAL

TYPE I

TYPE IV

TYPE II

TYPE V

TYPE III

TYPE VI

Conjoined london of
biceps and coracobrachialis

**Figure 5–3** Acromioclavicular injury types. Descriptions of each injury are given in **Table 5–3**. (From Rockwood Jr, CA, Matsen F III. The Shoulder. Philadelphia, PA: WB Saunders; 1990:423, Figure 12–13. Reprinted by permission.)

plane of motion. AC joint separations have been divided into six types (**Fig. 5–3**); each separation type typically correlates well with the constellation of the involved structures and the severity of the injury.[7–9] The continuum of injury starts with the AC ligaments and capsular complex, progresses to involve the CC ligaments, and continues with injury to the deltoid and trapezius muscles. These patterns of injury generally result in predictable positions of the clavicle.[1]

Tossy et al[7] and Allman[8] initially described the classification of AC injuries in the 1960s. This original classification system included types I, II, and III; however, in 1984 Rockwood[1] modified the classification system to include types IV, V, and VI (**Table 5–2**). AC joint injuries are approximately five times more common in men than in women, with type I and II injuries occurring twice as often as the more severe separations.[10] Grade III separations account for ~15% of all shoulder sprains in male hockey players.

**Table 5–2**   Classification of Injuries to the Acromioclavicular Joint

| Type | AC Ligament | CC Ligament | Fascia | Direction |
|------|-------------|-------------|--------|-----------|
| I | Sprain | Intact | Intact | Nondisplaced |
| II | Complete disruption | Sprain | Intact | <25% superior |
| III | Complete disruption | Complete disruption | Injury | 25–100% superior |
| IV | Complete disruption | Complete disruption | Detached | Posterior through trapezius |
| V | Complete disruption | Complete disruption | Detached | 100–300% superior |
| VI | Complete disruption | Complete disruption | Detached | Inferior to acromion or conoid |

*Source:* From Lemos MJ. The evaluation and treatment of the injured acromioclavicular joint in athletes. Am J Sports Med 1998;26:137–144. Reprinted by permission. AC, acromioclavicular; CC, coracoclavicular.

**Table 5–3**   Descriptions of AC Joint Injury

| | |
|--|--|
| Type I | A sprain to the AC ligament with no affect on the CC ligament or deltotrapezial fascia constitutes a type I injury. A type I injury has no displacement of the AC joint. |
| Type II | A complete disruption of the AC joint ligament complex and a sprain of the CC ligament with no effect on the deltotrapezial fascia constitute a type II injury. This injury will present visually with a <25% superior migration of the distal clavicle. |
| Type III | A complete disruption of the AC joint ligament complex, a complete disruption of the CC ligaments, and damage to the deltotrapezial fascia constitute a type III injury. This injury will present visually with a 25 to 100% superior migration of the distal clavicle. |
| Type IV | A complete disruption of both the AC and CC ligament complexes constitutes a type IV injury. The type IV injury will also present with a detached deltotrapezial fascia and a posteriorly migrated distal clavicle that penetrates through the trapezius. |
| Type V | A complete disruption of both the AC and CC ligament complexes as well as a detached deltotrapezial fascia and an exaggerated superior dislocation of the distal clavicle between 100 to 300% constitute a type IV injury. |
| Type VI | A complete disruption of the AC and CC ligament complexes as well as a detached delto-trapezial fascia constitute a type VI injury. The distal clavicle displaces inferiorly into the subacromial or subcoracoid position. |

## ◆ Examination and Presentation of Acromioclavicular Joint Injuries

Pain associated with an AC injury may be difficult to localize because of the complex sensory innervations of the joint.[2] The most important information during the examination process is gleaned by a thorough and extensive history. This information enables us to determine if the pain is a result of a separation or an ongoing degenerative process. Once it is determined that the pain is a result of an acute separation, further examination should address the level of pain, its location, and positions of relief. Each patient should also undergo a radiographic examination. The following are the general presentations of each separation type (**Table 5–4**):

*Type I*   With only a sprain of the AC joint ligaments, no joint deformity is apparent during physical or radiographic examination. Minimal tenderness and swelling may be present over the AC joint; however, the injury is inherently stable because the AC and CC ligaments are structurally intact.[1] The pain is generally self-limiting; however, patients will often report discomfort with full-arm abduction and flexion.

*Type II*   In type II injuries, the AC ligament complex is completely torn; therefore, vertical stability is maintained but sagittal stability is compromised.[1,11,12] On physical examination, like patients with type I injuries, patients with type II injuries present with pain as the primary symptom. Patients may present with a

**Table 5–4** Expected Initial Evaluation Presentation of Acromioclavicular Joint Injuries

|  | Type I | Type II | Type III |
|---|---|---|---|
| Appearance | Minimal swelling | Swelling | Swelling, step off |
| Radiology | Normal | Elevation <100% | Elevation >100% |
| Cosmesis | Not visible | May be visible | Step off deformity |
| Active ROM | Moderate pain; abduction | Significant pain | Significant pain |
| Passive ROM | Minimal pain | Moderate–severe pain | Severe pain |
| Resisted strength tests | Minimal pain; abd, ER | Moderate–severe pain | Severe pain |
| AC joint comp. test | Minimal pain | Moderate pain | Severe pain |
| Neurological | Normal | Normal | Normal |
| Joint play | Not remarkable | ↑ Posterior mobility | Excessive mobility |
| Palpation | Minimal/moderate over AC | Excessive pain | Minimal/moderate pain |

Abd, abduction; AC, acromioclavicular; ER, external rotation; ROM, range of motion.

mild superior migration of the distal clavicle, as compared with the acromion. This migration may be better appreciated by running a finger along the acromion medially to the AC joint.[2] Radiographic examination may also reveal this superior migration of the distal clavicle; however, the separation will be less than 100%. Patients may also present with minimal to moderate strength and ROM deficiencies. These deficiencies are typically secondary to the pain and not an alteration in the biomechanics of the AC joint.[13]

*Type III* In type III injuries, because the AC and CC ligaments are torn and the deltotrapezial fascia is detached, patients typically present with pain and an easily identifiable deformity called a *step-off deformity* (**Fig. 5–4**). Patients will typically present holding the arm in the adducted position to counteract the pain produced by the weight of the arm.[2] Upon radiographic evaluation, the clavicle appears elevated; however, further evaluation will show that the elevation is actually the inferior displacement of the acromion. The loss of the conoid and trapezoid ligaments will compromise the horizontal and vertical stability of the clavicle. Upon palpation, increased tenderness will be noted over the AC and CC joints, as well as excessive pain with any active arm movement.

*Type IV* In type IV injuries, a similar clinical presentation as the type III injury, is commonplace. The difference in presentation includes the level of pain (greater in type IV injuries) and the displacement of the clavicle. In type IV injuries, the distal clavicle may be displaced into the trapezius muscle. This displacement

into the muscle often causes the excessive pain that patients experience. The clavicular displacement is noted upon clinical presentation by a bump in the posterior skin of the shoulder. Radiographically, this can be confirmed by an axillary x-ray. It is also important to note the SC joint for an anteriorly dislocated clavicle. An anteriorly dislocated clavicle at the SC joint would reduce stress on the clavicle.[2]

*Type V* The type V injury is similar to a type III injury but more severe. Clinical presentation will include a severe shoulder droop, marked pain, and a CC distance increase up to three times.[2] However, the biggest difference from the type V and type III injury is the involvement of the deltoid and trapezial fascia. In the type V injury the fascia of the deltoid and trapezius is extensively stripped away from the bone. This

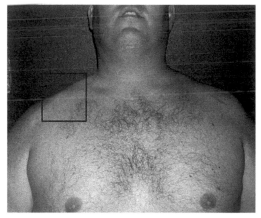

**Figure 5–4** Step-off deformity is a clinically distinguishable sign that is noticeable in type III acromioclavicular joint injuries.

condition is evident when the patient performs a shoulder shrug and the AC joint space does not reduce. Radiographically, the space between the clavicle and the acromion increases 100 to 300%.

*Type VI*   The type VI injury, although rare, is characterized by the inferior migration of the distal clavicle. Clinically, the acromion will be prominent on palpation with an obvious step down to the clavicle. It has been reported that occasional transient paresthesia accompanies this dislocation; however, it subsides with reduction.[14] Radiographically, the distal clavicle will be subluxed under the coracoid or acromion.

## ◆ Treatment of Acromioclavicular Injuries

Although the focus of this book is on nonoperative treatment approaches, it is difficult to discuss the AC joint without the often-debated surgical versus nonsurgical treatment approaches. The consensus is that types I and II AC joint separations are best treated with a conservative approach, whereas types IV through VI are best addressed with one of many surgical approaches; AC ligament repair, dynamic muscle transfer, CC ligament reconstruction, or CA ligament transfer. The greatest area of debate is the treatment decision making for type III AC joint injuries. In a literature review by Phillips et al,[15] 88% of surgically treated patients reported a satisfactory outcome; 87% of nonsurgically treated patients had a satisfactory outcome. A meta-analysis of the mix data from these studies showed no significant benefit from surgery.[15] There are over 32 methods of conservative treatment[16] and over 60 surgical procedures[17] that have been described to date; hence, this is a long-running debate. The most recent comparative studies between conservative and operative treatment for type III injuries have determined that nonoperative outcomes are as good, if not better, than current surgical procedures.[18–21] Conservatively treated patients have been found to return to work and activities faster than patients who received surgical treatments.[19] Considering outcome studies like these, a higher rate of patients will pursue a nonoperative approach to grade III AC joint injuries.

A properly designed rehab program for a nonoperative AC joint injury must be developed to address the functional needs of each specific patient. Professional and amateur athletes, the construction worker, as well as the sedentary desk worker can incur AC joint injuries. Each program must be designed with the patient's functional demands in mind. A well-designed program will address the five coexisting areas that make up the functionality of our upper extremities; range of motion (ROM), kinesthetic awareness, proprioception, neuromuscular control, and strength (**Fig. 5–5**). We will now review the goals, steps, and importance of each of the rehabilitation stages: the protective phase, the early mobility and stability phase, the late mobility and stability phase, and the return to activity phase.

### Treatment of Type I and II Injuries

The nonoperative treatment of a type I AC joint injury will often not be medically treated because patients typically ignore the injury. If medical care is provided, however, the primary treatment goals are to (1) regulate the pain response, (2) promote a healing environment as well as protect the damaged tissue, and (3) deter ROM loss. These objectives are inherent in the protective phase of rehabilitation.

Immediate care during the protective phase will include icing the injured area incrementally and positioning the arm in an arm sling

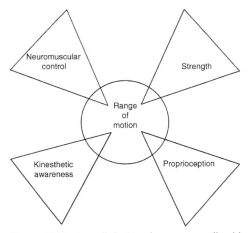

**Figure 5–5**   A well-designed program will address the five coexisting areas that make up the functionality of our upper extremities: range of motion, kinesthetic awareness, proprioception, neuromuscular control, and strength.

for up to 1 week. Passive or active assisted ROM exercises are recommended during this period to create nourishment to the articular cartilage and promote collagen synthesis and organization. These may include early supine IR and ER motions beginning at the neutral position and progressing to the scapular plane. It is important that patients use their pain as a guide to ROM exercises. Excessive stressing of the damaged tissues may initiate an excessive inflammatory response.

Early treatment (the protective phase) of a type II injury is important because of the complete disruption of the AC joint ligament. Although the CC ligaments are still intact, the horizontal and axial stability of the AC joint is compromised because of the loss of the AC ligament. To maximize the healing and essential scarring to realign the AC joint, it is recommended that the patient wear a Kenny Howard sling or an AirCast AC Joint Sports Sling (Aircast Corp., Summit, NJ) (**Fig. 5–6**) for up to 3 weeks. If an AC joint sling is not available, for the patient's comfort a standard shoulder sling should be worn for up to 3 weeks. During this phase of the rehabilitation, the application of ice is recommended to control swelling and to alleviate pain. The important steps taken in the protective phase include (1) educating patients on their injury and rehabilitation,

(2) maintaining ROM, and (3) diminishing pain levels.

For the other three phases of rehabilitation, we follow the guidelines for a type III, however progress at a faster pace; we sometimes progress through a stage in a day or two. Patients typically return to activities and sports within 2 to 4 weeks, once full ROM and strength are normal. For contact sports like football and hockey, a protective pad placed over the AC joint is recommended to add protection to the joint (**Fig. 5–7**).

## Treatment of Type III Injuries

### Protective Phase

A type III injury is addressed as in a type I/II injury; however, during a type III injury to the AC joint, patients will have a noticeable deformity immediately and will generally have an elevated level of pain because of the structures compromised. With the disruption of the AC ligaments, the CC ligaments, and the possibility of fascia damage to the trapezius or deltoid, patients will present with excessive pain that must be addressed during this protective

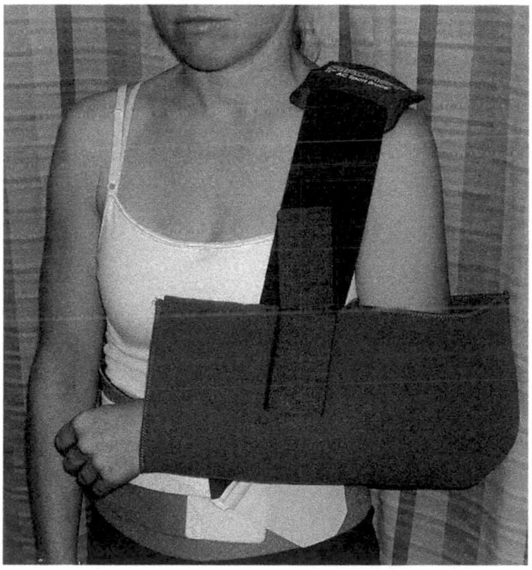

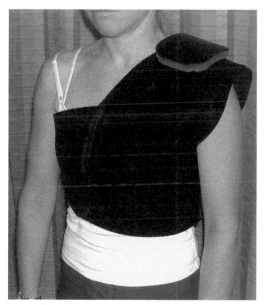

**Figure 5–6**  An AirCast acromioclavicular Joint Sports Sling is often prescribed to approximate the injured joint and relieve the weighted arm from distraction.

**Figure 5–7**  A protective acromioclavicular joint pad, the Sully AC (The Saunders Group Chaska, MN) is often prescribed for contact sport athletes when returning to their sport.

phase. During this stage, the primary treatment goals are to (1) protect the damaged tissue and promote a healing environment, (2) deter ROM, and (3) regulate the pain response.

During this protective phase, the patient would have the arm immobilized in a Kenny Howard sling or an AirCast AC Joint Sports Sling to approximate the separated ends of the distal clavicle and the acromion. During the protective phase, active assisted ROM can begin once the pain and swelling have minimized. These include internal rotation (IR) and external rotation (ER) at the neutral position with a T-bar or cane (**Fig. 5–8**). While performing this exercise it is important to maintain the humerus in a neutral position with minimal extension. This can be accomplished by supporting the distal humerus with a towel roll or pillow. Glenohumeral (GH) extension will put undo stress on the AC joint causing pain. At this point, it is also important to minimize the level of abduction and flexion to 30 to 40 degrees[22] to minimize AC joint compression. Inman et al[23] reported that the AC joint motion occurs during the first 30 degrees of abduction and above 135 degrees of elevation. Although the AC and CC ligaments are completely disrupted with a type III injury, the upward rotation of the clavicle may still cause pain with passive ROM activities due to joint compression. By performing ranges of flexion and abduction below 40 degrees scapular motion is minimized, which in turn decreases the chances of joint compression or grading.

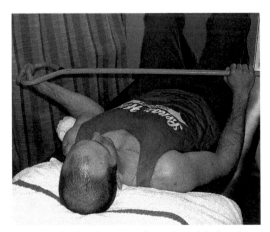

**Figure 5–8** Passive external rotation with the glenohumeral joint at 0 degrees of abduction.

Excessive scapular motion will cause increased stress to the AC joint, inhibiting healing. For this reason, patients are often instructed to use pain as their guide. ROM can be progressed within pain tolerance.

During this stage, the reduction of pain and inflammation is addressed. In addition to nonsteroidal antiinflammatory drugs (NSAIDs) or pain medication prescribed by the doctor, certain modalities may assist with alleviating pain and swelling. Pain reducing modalities may include ice, high-volt stimulation, high-intensity stimulation, and transcutaneous neuromuscular stimulation. Utilizing gentle joint mobilizations to the AC, SC, and GH joints may also help neuromodulate pain by stimulating the type I and type II joint receptors. The introduction of pendulums may also assist with alleviating pain and causing some joint receptor stimulation. Pendulums have been shown to produce very little muscular activity[24] and may be considered to be a safe exercise during this period. Surprisingly, unpublished cadaveric data from our institute have shown that gravity distraction of the GH joint (as with pendulums) does not cause marked stress across the CC ligaments. With this in mind, initiating pendulums on a physioball in a patient's rehabilitation program may take stress off the healing ligaments and reduce pain (**Fig. 5–9**).

Applying ice to the affected area can be the easiest and one of the most beneficial treatments that can be utilized at home and in the clinic. We recommend that the patient apply ice for pain and swelling three to five times a day during this protective phase for up to 15 minutes for each application. We have also had some success utilizing high-volt stimulation in the event of excessive swelling. Currently, the 300 PV unit from Empi (St. Paul, MN) has given our clinic the ability to utilize the high-volt setting as well as controlling the unit to perform high-intensity electrical stimulation or "noxious-level stimulation." This type of stimulation is believed to effect pain amelioration by an endorphin-mediated mechanism. The stimulation is applied on the joint, over noncontractile tissues (**Fig. 5–10**). At higher stimulation levels, all types of fibers in the peripheral nerve are activated, and this painful stimulus likely modulates pain by an endorphin-mediated mechanism.[25] This type of stimulation is not tolerated well by patients with a low-level pain

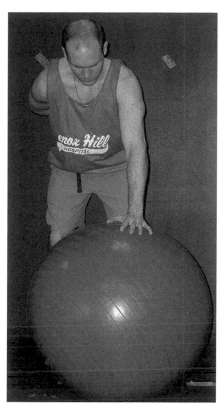

**Figure 5–9** Initiating pendulums on a physioball may take stress off the healing ligaments.

threshold; patients must also be closely monitored for possible skin irritations. The current parameters for this treatment are 12 seconds on, 8 seconds off for 15 minutes with a 2-second ramp time; phase duration should be 400 μs

and the frequency should be set at 50 pps. Utilizing these settings, the stimulation should be raised to maximally tolerated levels.

Taping of the acutely injured AC joint has been documented to relieve pain and enable a greater active ROM.[26] Treatment at our clinic utilizes the taping technique described by Shamus and Shamus[26] to enhance the treatment of acutely injured AC joints (**Fig. 5–11**) (**Table 5–5**). By utilizing the tape to approximate the joint and add stability, patients will experience a marked decrease in pain, muscle guarding, and spasms. By breaking the muscle spasm cycle and decreasing the pain, patients are able to increase their strength, ROM, and function at a faster rate. Taping, however, should only be used as an adjunct to the treatment of AC joint injuries and not as a replacement for therapeutic exercises. It is believed that excessive taping may alter (inhibit or excite) muscular firing patterns.

The patient's key objectives in the protective phase are (1) to adhere to precautions, (2) to comply with a home exercise program, (3) to maintain the current ROM, and (4) to decrease pain.

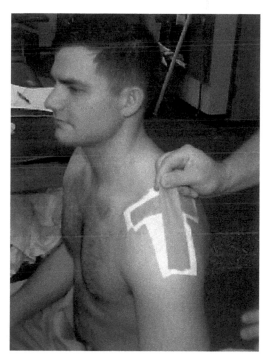

**Figure 5–11** Taping may help stabilize and support the healing ligaments; see **Table 5–5** for taping instructions.

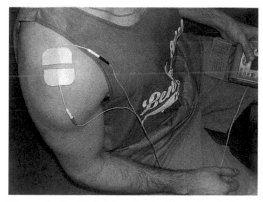

**Figure 5–10** High-intensity electrical stimulation or "noxious-level stimulation" setup.

**Table 5–5**   Taping the Acromioclavicular Joint

1. Remove the sling and expose the shoulder for taping.
2. A skin preparation is applied if the patient has a known sensitivity to tape. (Taping not recommended for patients with known allergies to tape)
3. Hypafix tape (Smith & Nephew Healthcare Ltd., Hull, UK) is measured and cut to fit from:
   a. The insertion of the middle deltoid inferiorly to 2.5 cm proximal to the AC joint superiorly
   b. The coracoid process of the scapula anteriorly to the spine of the scapula posteriorly
4. These pieces of tape are then laid gently on the skin in respective order.
5. Leukotape (3M, Maplewood, MN) is then measured and cut to form two pieces 0.5 cm shorter than the first piece of Hypafix tape and two pieces 0.5 cm shorter than the second piece of Hypafix tape.
6. The first piece of Leukotape is anchored at the insertion of the deltoid and pulled superiorly with a considerable amount of force so that the arm is firmly supported. At the same time, the joint should be approximated with the other hand by supporting the elbow and pushing the humerus superiorly. The patient's shoulder must be relaxed. Wrinkles in the Hypafix tape should appear if this part of the procedure is done correctly. Be careful not to tape the upper trapezius muscle belly because not only does it interfere with muscle recruitment, it is very uncomfortable.
7. The second piece of Leukotape is started over the coracoid process and pulled posteriorly to secure it near the spine of the scapula. This piece of tape should minimize superior translation of the distal end of the clavicle and act as an anchor for the first piece of tape.
8. Steps 6 and 7 are repeated to provide extra reinforcement and to extend the tape's effectiveness over time.
9. Patients are instructed to monitor the area for signs of redness and to remove the tape if any irritation occurs. For tape-sensitive persons, it is recommended that the tape be worn for 1 hour the first day, 2 hours the second day, etc.

*Source:* From Shamus JL, Shamus EC. A taping technique for the treatment of acromioclavicular joint sprains: a case report. J Orthop Sports Phys Ther 1997;25:390–394. Reprinted by permission.

### Early Mobility and Stability Phase

The early mobility and stability phase is designed to enhance ROM following the immbilization period. The concept of "linkage" between other joints must be considered while addressing the mobility and stability of the surrounding joints. During this stage, treatment goals for a type III injury are (1) to address ROM issues, (2) to attend to scapular and proximal weakness, and (3) to initiate rotator cuff strengthening.

Advancing pain-free ROM during this phase is essential to progressing toward full ROM by the next phase. Patients are encouraged to continue with active assisted ROM exercises within a pain-free range. Utilizing an L-bar or a cane will enable the patient to direct the range actively and progressively. At this time, regaining flexion is highly encouraged, and external rotation is advanced gradually from a neutral position to the scapular plane. Once active assisted or passive ROM reaches ~130 degrees of pain-free flexion, active motion can begin. Active flexion is recommended to 90 degrees or to the level of initiation of altered scapulothoracic (ST) motion. Active IR and ER can also begin once pain-free passive ER reaches ~45 degrees in the scapular plane and IR of 50 degrees. At this time, the mobility of the SC joint and ST joint are addressed and mobilized if indicated. Once mobility of these proximal joints is obtained, manual GH stabilization is initiated.

The deltoid and upper trapezius muscles are both considered secondary stabilizers of the AC joint; as such, these muscles need to regain their structural stability. Submaximal isometrics for all deltoid heads as well as the upper trapezius are an important start to strengthening during this early stability stage. To initiate rotator cuff stability, submaximal alternating isometrics and rhythmic stabilization at neutral are optimal techniques (**Fig. 5–12A,B**). The initiation of these therapeutic exercises must be guided by the patient's pain. Because of the compromised joint integrity, altered lines of pull from muscle contractions may cause pain during early tissue healing. Next, the entire shoulder complex should undergo isometric strengthening. Primary strengthening during this stage should only include submaximal isometric

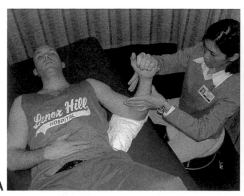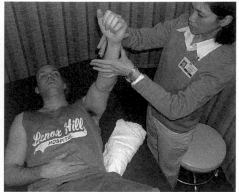

A

B

**Figure 5–12** **(A)** Alternating isometrics at 45 degrees abduction for internal and external rotators. **(B)** Alternating isometrics in the scapular plane. These can be progressed by having patients close their eyes to eliminate visual feedback.

strengthening to negate scapular motion. Progressing from manual isometric contractions to manual assisted isometric contractions with the physioball will add an early, low-level closed kinetic chain contraction. These ball contraction exercises, as well as manual isometric contraction exercises, should also promote a proprioceptive awareness by the patient. This is done by challenging patients, in a systematic pattern to watch and look away from the exercise as well as close their eyes during the exercise (**Fig. 5–13**).

Standard isometric contractions can be advanced to interactive isometric contractions utilizing Theraband (Hygenic Corp., Akron, OH). Interactive isometric contractions offer another way to control the isometric resistance offered. For the flexors one end of the Theraband is secured to a stable surface while the other end is held by the patient or secured to the patient's wrist (**Fig. 5–14A,B**). The patient faces away from the stable surface and then begins to slowly step away while maintaining the arm in a neutral position. The further distance away from the fixed band, the greater the stabilizing force that is needed. Altering the band color or the distance from the stable surface can regulate the resistance. Interactive isometric contractions can be used for all the prime muscles of the shoulder as well as the GH rotators (**Fig. 5–14C,D**).

Kinesthetic awareness training can also be introduced at this time. Considering the altered kinematics and loading patterns[12,27,28] associated with damaged AC and CC ligaments, apparent impaired proprioception will manifest. During the early mobility and stability phase, introductory joint position, mirror position, and reposition senses can be retrained with little to no impact on the healing tissue. Lying supine with arms in the scapular plane, patients are instructed to externally rotate their arms bilaterally at the same rate, through the same ROM. Having patients progress from eyes open to eyes closed will allow them to practice with

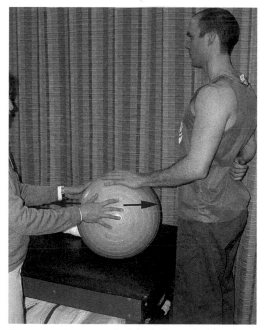

**Figure 5–13** Resisted physioball isometric contractions will add a low-level closed kinetic chain component as well as early proprioceptive training.

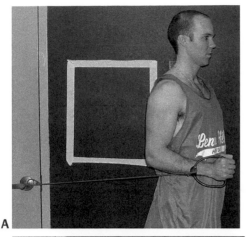

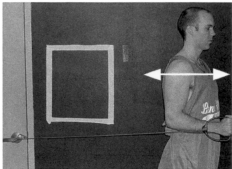

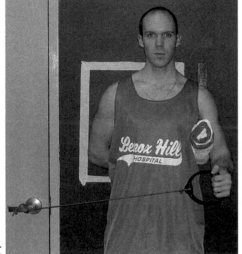

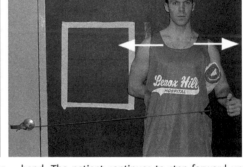

**Figure 5–14** **(A)** In initiating interactive isometrics for the flexors, stabilize the glenohumeral (GH) joint at neutral and flex the patient's elbow to 90 degrees. The patient grasps the T-band and pulls up the slack of the band. **(B)** Continuing to stabilize the GH joint at neutral, the patient steps forward to increase the tension on the band. The patient continues to step forward until the proper resistance is felt, then back steps to the original starting point and returns. **(C)** Initiating interactive isometrics for the external rotators. **(D)** Stepping out to tighten the band and activate the external rotators.

and without their visual sense. Patients then progress to positioning their involved shoulder in a "mirror" position of the noninvolved static shoulder. The success of these training techniques can be documented by utilizing goniometry or digital levels (**Fig. 5–15**).

Early strengthening of the scapular muscles helps to deter altered ST movement during the latter stages of rehabilitation. We initiate the scapular strengthening in the same manner as in the treatment of an early upper-extremity injury, but with consideration of the muscular balance between the serratus anterior and the lower trapezius. These two muscle groups work together to perform an upward and outward rotation of the scapula. In the side-lying position, manual resistance can be given to the scapula to resist elevation, depression, protraction, and retraction. During these exercises, attention must be given to the AC joint. Because of the scapular attachment to the clavicle, some manual resistance exercises may put stress on the joint. If pain is noted, the strain placed on the joint should be reduced. In some instances, by manually approximating the joint, pain can be eliminated using these scapular exercises.

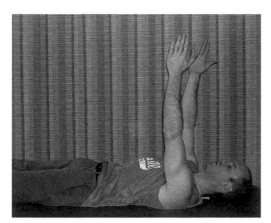

**Figure 5–15** Joint positioning and mirror repositioning for flexion can be an integral part of retraining proprioception.

The patient's key objectives in the early mobility and stability phase are (1) to achieve within 80% of full PROM for all planes of motion, (2) to experience minimal pain and tenderness on palpation of the AC joint, and (3) to show no greater than a 30% strength deficit in IR and ER at neutral when measured with a hand-held dynamometer. Because the upper trapezius is a difficult muscle to test with a hand-held dynamometer, a manual muscle test rating of 4/5 is needed to advance to the advanced mobility and stability phase.

### Advanced Mobility and Stability Phase

Once a patient has reached the advanced mobility and stability phase, the goals shift to (1) regaining full passive pain-free ROM, (2) regaining 85% of active pain-free ROM, and (3) normalizing strength. During this stage, focus is spent on actively strengthening the prime GH movers through the arc of motion; progressing the rotational strength toward the more functional position in the scapular plane; and eventually progressing to 90 degrees of shoulder abduction and 90 degrees of elbow flexion for rotational training.

Isotonic training begins with strengthening of the shoulder rotators at 0 degrees of shoulder abduction. Strengthening the external rotators is not only important for stabilization of the GH joint but also plays an integral part in developing an approximation force on the shoulder

during the overhead throwing motion.[29] Setting up an early program of proper ER strengthening will set a solid foundation from which the whole rehabilitation process can progress. Reinold et al[30] found that performing a 10-repetition ("rep") maximum, side-lying ER (**Fig. 5–16**) at 0 degrees of abduction activated the infraspinatus to 62% of maximum voluntary isometric contraction (MVIC), and the teres minor was activated 67% of MVIC. Townsend et al[31] found similar increased activity in the infraspinatus and teres minor during side-lying external rotation (SLER). SLER may be initiated early in the program or added later, but it provides the base for isotonic strengthening of the external rotators. Rotational strengthening must be rapidly progressed to the scapular plane to advance functional strength. To strengthen the shoulder rotators, a proper strength-training program includes the use of weights, resistive bands, manual resistance, and isokinetic exercises (if available) (**Fig. 5–17**).

Isotonic strengthening of the deltoids should be initiated in the scapular position prior to starting sagittal and frontal plane strengthening. Once patients can elevate their shoulder pain free and without an altered ST motion to 90 degrees, sagittal and frontal plane strengthening can begin. As with the shoulder rotators, a spectrum of strengthening methods (**Fig. 5–18**) is recommended to address deltoid weakness. Considering the secondary stabilizing features of the deltoid and trapezius muscle to the AC joint, placement of weights and resistive force

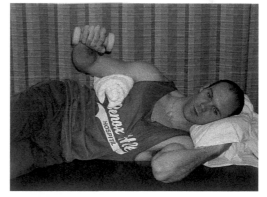

**Figure 5–16** Side-lying external rotation is an easy, yet effective way to activate the glenohumeral external rotators.

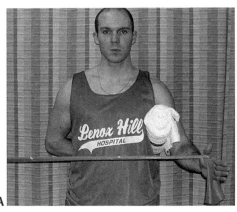 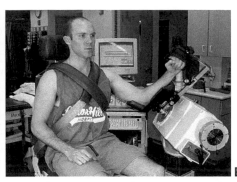

A B

**Figure 5–17** **(A)** External rotation can be progressed through the spectrum of band resistances. **(B)** Utilizing isokinetics in the safe 30 degree/30 degree/30 degree[38] position will enable training of the glenohumeral rotators through the isokinetic speed spectrum.

should be considered when training the trapezius muscle. Patients should *not* hold dumbbells or cuff weights during shrugging exercises. This distractive weight may add undue stress to the healing joint and cause excessive irritation if full scarring has not occurred. Manual resistance to the shoulder or approximating the injury with Theraband while performing shrugs is a safe alternative (**Fig. 5–19**).

The effect of roller board training has been well established in the lower extremities.[32] Utilizing a progression of roller board and perturbation training, 92% of anterior cruciate ligament (ACL) deficient patients returned to full activity. Our institute has taken this theory of roller board training to the upper extremity and has developed a progressive upper-extremity

training program to regain proprioception and strength. Although the program can usually begin as soon as deltoid isometric exercises are initiated, we feel it should not be initiated with patients who have AC joint separations until the advanced mobility and stability phase. The progressive program has six stages with three training sessions per stage (**Table 5–6**). The stages include (1) the neutral stage with arm at the side holding onto the roller board; (2) the incline stage with the arm at ~50 degrees of flexion with the roller board on an incline; (3) the elbow flexion stage with the GH joint at neutral and the elbow flexed to 90 degrees holding onto the board against the wall; (4) the

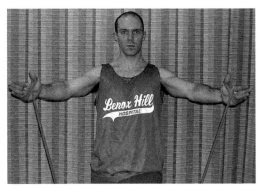 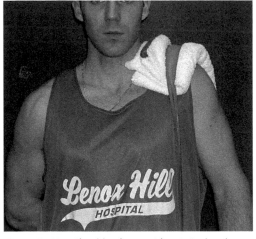

**Figure 5–18** Deltoid strengthening can be addressed through resistive band training, initiating strengthening in the scapular plane.

**Figure 5–19** Shoulder shrugs with resistive bands may be a safe alternative to shrugs with shoulder distraction.

**Table 5–6**  Upper Extremity Roller Board Training*

| Position | Session 1 | Sessions 2 and 3 | Training Time |
|---|---|---|---|
| 1. Neutral position | Watching board; straight plane movements | Eyes closed; random straight plane movements | 30–40 seconds per set |
| 2. Incline position | Looking straight ahead; straight plane movements | Eyes closed; diagonal movements | |
| 3. Elbow flexed position | Eyes closed; straight plane movements | Looking straight ahead; straight plane and diagonals | |
| 4. Scaption position | Watching board; diagonal movements | Eyes closed; straight plane diagonals as previous; random forces | |
| 5. 150 degree position | Looking straight ahead; diagonal movements | As previous; random forces and time of perturbation | |
| 6. 90 degree/ 90 degree position | Eyes closed; diagonal movements | Eyes closed; straight plane and diagonal movements | |

*Each training position has three treatment sessions. Once these treatment sessions are complete, the treatment advances to the next treatment position. This continues until the entire progression is complete.

scaption stage with the arm at 90 degrees of flexion in the scapular plane holding onto the board against the wall; (5) 150 degrees of shoulder elevation; and finally (6) the functional stage with the GH joint at 90 degrees of abduction and the elbow flexed to 90 degrees holding onto the board (**Fig. 5–20A–D**). Alterations to each stage are based on visual input, direction of perturbation, speed and pressure of perturbation. Although we have yet to publish any studies on the strength and proprioceptive outcomes of upper-extremity roller board training, clinically we have had favorable results utilizing this training in conjunction with standard therapeutic exercises.

Considering the deltoid is a secondary stabilizer to the AC joint as well as a prime mover of the GH joint, the general force couples between the deltoid and the rotator cuff are an important aspect of shoulder strength that must be considered. To address this clinically, we utilize Bodyblade (Hymanson, Inc., Playa del Rey, CA) and Theraband flexbar training to incorporate these force couples into the training regimen. Bodyblade and Theraband training for AC joint patients should address the patient's ability to oscillate the blade horizontally and vertically while maintaining the shoulder at 90 degrees of flexion in the scapular plane (**Fig. 5–21A,B**). Once these oscillations are maintained in a rhythmic motion for up to 1 minute, the patient should be challenged outside of the scapular plane. Other recommended positions include 90 degrees of abduction, 120 to 150 degrees of flexion, or oscillations through a set ROM.

Closed kinetic chain exercises can also be initiated during this stage. We recommend beginning these with simple wall pushups in a controlled range to prevent excessive shearing of the AC joint. Once these are mastered, incorporate the physioball into the wall pushup. Use caution when guiding a patient in any closed kinetic chain position, especially the pushup position. With a disrupted AC joint, the distal end of the clavicle is free to move posteriorly, and is thus unable to fully provide the stable construct needed to resist the forces induced during a bench press or pushup.[33] Consider the patient's pain and degree of joint grating when guiding these closed chain exercises. Once patients can comfortably handle the quadruped position or the pushup ready position, the use of the Fitter (Fitter International, Inc., Alberta, Calgary, Canada) can be used to work on GH co-contraction while in a closed chain position (**Fig. 5–22**). Utilizing time bouts of horizontal or vertical weight shifting, the patient will gain confidence to perform physioball walkouts. Physioball walkouts incorporate not only upper extremity stability but also the utilization of core muscles for stability (**Fig. 5–23**).

Finally, the importance of the scapular musculature, although not fully understood, must

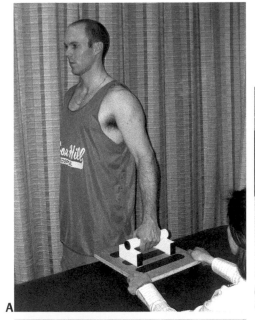

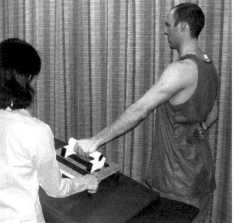

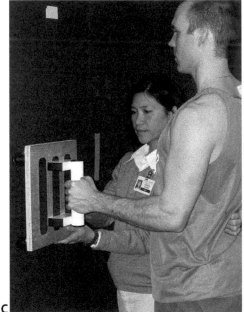

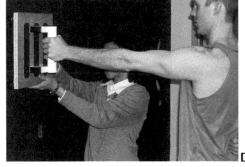

**Figure 5–20** **(A)** Roller board training level I: glenohumeral joint at 0 degrees. **(B)** Roller board training level II: glenohumeral joint at 45 degrees. **(C)** Roller board training level III: glenohumeral joint at 0 degrees, elbow flexed to 90 degrees. **(D)** Roller board training level IV: glenohumeral joint at 90 degrees in scapular plane.

be addressed when we consider that proximal stability will offer distal mobility for our patients. Clinically, we address any scapular weakness with our "prone program." Our prone program is based on electromyogram (EMG) studies investigating upper-extremity strengthening exercises.[31,34,35] The exercises are designed to address each of the scapular muscles that stabilize the scapula to the body. Each exercise is performed in the prone

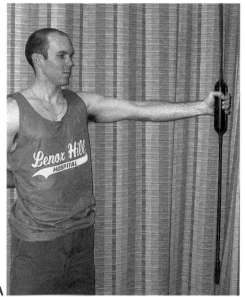
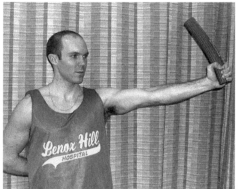

A                     B

**Figure 5–21** **(A)** BodyBlade oscillations at 90 degrees of flexion in the scapular plane. **(B)** Therabar oscillations >90 degrees of flexion in the scapular plane.

position and can be performed unilaterally or bilaterally if positioned properly. They include horizontal abduction with IR, horizontal abduction with ER, shoulder flexion in the scapular plane to 150 degrees, and 90/90 degree rows with external rotation (**Fig. 5–24A–D**).

We have described many exercises in this chapter that we expect the experienced therapist would incorporate during each phase of a patient's recovery. A few exercises, however, are contraindicated in the rehabilitation of a patient with AC joint separation. Upright rows are an exercise performed to activate deltoids and gain upper-extremity strength; this exercise, although it targets the muscle, can cause excessive grating and compression in the AC joint of a healthy individual. Its effects on a

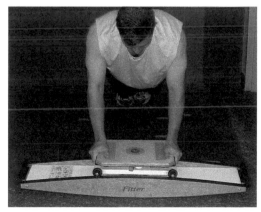

**Figure 5–22** Fitter training to promote advanced closed kinetic chain stability. Timed intervals of 10 to 15 seconds to begin are recommended—working up to longer times for endurance.

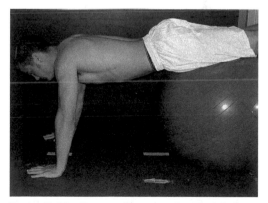

**Figure 5–23** Prone walkouts on the physioball are another way to train advanced closed kinetic chain strengthening while addressing the core musculature.

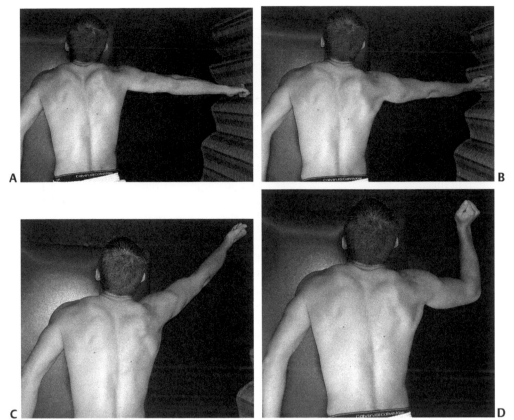

**Figure 5–24** **(A)** Prone horizontal abduction with internal rotation. **(B)** Prone horizontal abduction with external rotation. **(C)** Prone flexion in the scapular plane to horizontal position. **(D)** Prone scapular retraction with external rotation in the 90 degree/90 degree position.

damaged AC joint are even worse. Full-weighted dips are another exercise that should not be incorporated in the rehabilitation program of most shoulder patients, especially those with AC joint separations. Unpublished data from our institute revealed that in cadaveric AC joints, excessive force was generated through the CC ligament during GH extension. Although the CC ligament is already disrupted in type III injuries, our data suggest that excessive forces are placed through the AC joint during extension. Full weight-bearing dips place the GH joint into extension; therefore, we do not recommend performing this exercise at any stage of the rehabilitation process.

The key objectives of the patient's in the late mobility and stability phase are (1) a return of full passive ROM, (2) the ability to lift 5 lb in the scapular plane to shoulder level, and (3) achieving a <30% strength deficit throughout all muscle groups in the upper extremity. Once these objectives are accomplished, the patient can begin the return to activity phase.

### Return to Activity Phase

During this phase, the patient's goal is to possess the appropriate ROM, strength, and functional capabilities to perform primary activities. Hence, strength training is designed to incorporate plyometric activities, functional activities, and normalization of functional position strength deficits.

The literature has well established that there are little to no strength deficits in conservatively treated grade III AC joint separations.[33,36] Schlegel et al[33] recently determined that there were no isokinetic strength differences in males or females for flexion, extension, abduction, adduction, IR, or ER. This study did find a statistical difference of 17% in the bench press strength of the involved limb versus the noninvolved limb. Interestingly, this finding correlated with patients' subjective reports of weakness with maximal lifting. This study as well as others[19–22] provides evidence that despite a traumatic event to the shoulder, in due time, shoulder strength does normalize to that of the noninvolved side.

Proprioceptive neuromuscular facilitation (PNF) exercises are an essential functional component in this final phase of rehabilitation. Although we may incorporate some PNF techniques earlier in the rehabilitation process, the functional motions of D1 and D2 should be stressed during these stages. These techniques should not only be performed manually with the patient in a supine position, but the patient should also use resistive bands and isokinetic exercises (if available) (**Fig. 5–25A,B**). In utilizing all of these components, the therapist addresses the entire spectrum of exercise training to ensure the return of functional strength and stabilization.

Plyometric training is also an essential functional component of treatment, which needs to be addressed prior to discharge. Plyometrics for the upper extremity generate rapid and powerful muscular contractions in response to a dynamic stretch-inducing load to a muscle or group of muscles. Plyometrics can train the entire neuromuscular system, utilizing the principles of stored elastic energy to use strength as quickly and forcefully as possible. The myostatic stretch reflex develops stored elastic potential. If the exercise movement is slow, such as in weightlifting, the energy is dissipated and nonproductive. However, with rapid movement, this stored elastic energy can generate a force greater than that of the concentric contraction of the muscle alone. Plyometrics employ the principles of progressive loading with the ultimate goal of power development. Utilizing a trampoline will increase the EMG activity and elevate the level of eccentric loading of the shoulder rotators.[37] Plyometric training should include a progression of bilateral ball tosses, unilateral internal rotation tosses at neutral, unilateral posterior cuff tosses, unilateral functional 90/90 (90 degrees of abduction and 90 degrees of ER) position tosses for internal and external rotators (**Fig. 5–26**).

Prior to full return to activity, contact athletes like football and hockey players may want to consider protective equipment like a shoulder girdle or donut pad to protect the AC joint. These protective devices offer extra padding and resistance from compressing the involved joint. Although these devices do not guarantee against further AC joint damage,

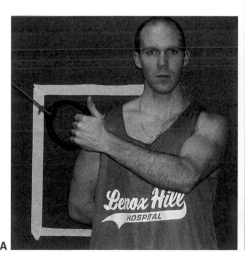
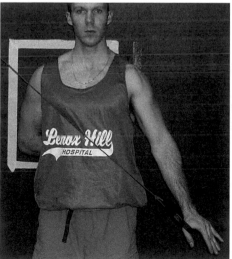

A B

**Figure 5–25** **(A)** Proprioceptive neuromuscular facilitation (PNF) exercise, D2 starting position utilizing resistive bands. **(B)** PNF D2 finishing position utilizing resistive bands.

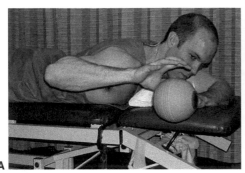
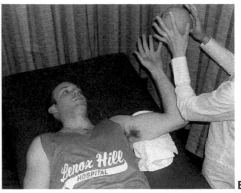

**Figure 5–26** **(A)** Prone plyometrics for external rotators; while positioning the arm in the 90/90 position, the patient releases the plyoball and quickly grasps it before it falls to the ground.

**(B)** Supine plyometrics for the internal rotators; while positioning the arm in the 90 degree/90 degree position, the patient catches and immediately tosses the plyoball back to the therapist.

they offer a level of protection that would not have been there otherwise.

The patient's key objectives in the return to activity phase include (1) full pain-free active and passive ROM, (2) normalized strength throughout ROM, (3) <10% strength deficits in all muscle groups with isokinetic and/or hand-held dynamometer testing, and (4) normalized closed kinetic chain testing.

## ◆ Summary

Anatomy and knowledge regarding the biomechanics of the AC joint and its supportive structures, as well as a complete understanding of the injury classification, provide the essential background for the patient with an AC joint injury. Designing a rehabilitation program that includes interventions to address ROM, neuromuscular control, and both proprioception and kinesthetic awareness is warranted to return full function via nonoperative treatment.

## References

1. Rockwood CA Jr, Williams G, Young DC. Injuries to the acromioclavicular joint. In: Rockwood CA Jr, Green DP, Bucholz RW, Heckman JD, eds. Fractures in Adults. 4th ed. Philadelphia: Lippincott-Raven; 1996: 1341–1413

2. Dumonski M, Mazzocca AD, Rios C, Romeo AA, Arciero RA. Evaluation and management of acromioclavicular joint injuries. Am J Orthop 2004;33: 526–532

3. Codman E. The Shoulder. Malabar, FL: Robert E. Krieger Publishing Co.; 1934

4. Salter EG Jr, Nasca RJ, Shelley BS. Anatomical observations on the acromioclavicular joint and supporting ligaments. Am J Sports Med 1987;15:199–206

5. Fukuda K, Craig EV, An KN, Cofield RH, Chao EY. Biomechanical study of the ligamentous system of the acromioclavicular joint. J Bone Joint Surg Am 1986;68:434–440

6. Debski RE, Parsons IM, Woo SL, Fu FH. Effect of capsular injury on acromioclavicular joint mechanics. J Bone Joint Surg Am 2001;83-A:1344–1351

7. Tossy JD, Mead NC, Sigmond HM. Acromioclavicular separations: useful and practical classification for treatment. Clin Orthop Relat Res 1963;28: 111–119

8. Allman FL Jr. Fractures and ligamentous injuries of the clavicle and its articulation. J Bone Joint Surg Am 1967;49:774–784

9. Jerosch J, Filler T, Peuker E, Greig M, Siewering U. Which stabilization technique corrects anatomy best in patients with AC-separation? an experimental study. Knee Surg Sports Traumatol Arthrosc 1999;7: 365–372

10. Lemos MJ. The evaluation and treatment of the injured acromioclavicular joint in athletes. Am J Sports Med 1998;26:137–144

11. Debski RE, Parsons IM, Woo SL, Fu FH. Effect of capsular injury on acromioclavicular joint mechanics. J Bone Joint Surg Am 2001;83-A:1344–1351

12. Lee KW, Debski RE, Chen CH, Woo SL, Fu FH. Functional evaluation of the ligaments at the acromioclavicular joint during anteroposterior and superoinferior translation. Am J Sports Med 1997; 25:858–862

13. Bradley JP, Elkousy H. Decision making: operative versus nonoperative treatment of acromioclavicular joint injuries. Clin Sports Med 2003;22:277–290

14. McPhee IB. Inferior dislocation of the outer end of the clavicle. J Trauma 1980;20:709–710

15. Phillips AM, Smart C, Groom AF. Acromioclavicular dislocation: conservative or surgical therapy. Clin Orthop Relat Res 1998;353:10–17

16. Jacobs B, Wade PA. Acromioclavicular-joint injury: an end-result study. J Bone Joint Surg Am 1966;48: 475–486

17. Cook DA, Heiner JP. Acromioclavicular joint injuries. Orthop Rev 1990;19:510–516

18. Imatani RJ, Hanlon JJ, Cady GW. Acute, complete acromioclavicular separation. J Bone Joint Surg Am 1975;57:328–332

19. Larsen E, Bjerg-Nielsen A, Christensen P. Conservative or surgical treatment of acromioclavicular dislocation: a prospective, controlled. randomized study. J Bone Joint Surg Am 1986;68:552–555

20. Galpin RD, Hawkins RJ, Grainger RW. A comparative analysis of operative versus nonoperative treatment of grade III acromioclavicular separations. Clin Orthop Relat Res 1985;193:150–155

21. MacDonald PB, Alexander MJ, Frejuk J, Johnson GE. Comprehensive functional analysis of shoulders following complete acromioclavicular separation. Am J Sports Med 1988;16(5):475–480

22. Gladstone J, Wilk K, Andrews J. Nonoperative treatment of acromioclavicular joint injuries. Oper Tech Sports Med 1997;5:78–87

23. Inman VT, Saunders JB, Abbott LC. Observations of the function of the shoulder joint. J Bone Joint Surg 1944. 26:1–30

24. McCann PD, Wootten ME, Kadaba MP, Bigliani LU. A kinematic and electromyographic study of shoulder rehabilitation exercises. Clin Orthop Relat Res 1993;288:179–188

25. Robinson AJ, Snyder-Mackler L. Electrical Stimulation for Pain Modulation. In: Butler J. Clinical Electrophysiology; Electrotherapy and Electrophysiologic Testing. 2nd ed. Baltimore: Williams & Wilkins; 1995:281–332

26. Shamus JL, Shamus EC. A taping technique for the treatment of acromioclavicular joint sprains: a case study. J Orthop Sports Phys Ther 1997;25:390–394

27. Costic RS, Jari R, Rodosky MW, Debski RE. Joint compression alters the kinematics and loading patterns of the intact and capsule-transected AC joint. J Orthop Res 2003;21:379–385

28. Deshmukh AV, Wilson DR, Zilberfarb JL, Perlmutter GS. Stability of acromioclavicular joint reconstruction: biomechanical testing of various surgical techniques in a cadaveric model. Am J Sports Med 2004; 32:1492–1498

29. Fleisig GS, Barrentine SW, Escamilla RF, Andrews JR. Biomechanics of overhand throwing with implications for injuries. Sports Med 1996;21:421–437

30. Reinold MM, Wilk KE, Fleisig GS, et al. Electromyographic analysis of the rotator cuff and deltoid musculature during common shoulder external rotation exercises. J Orthop Sports Phys Ther 2004; 34:385–394

31. Townsend H, Jobe FW, Pink M, Perry J. Electromyographic analysis of the glenohumeral muscles during a baseball rehabilitation program. Am J Sports Med 1991;19:264–272

32. Fitzgerald GK, Axe MJ, Snyder-Mackler L. The efficacy of perturbation training in nonoperative anterior cruciate ligament rehabilitation programs for physical active individuals. Phys Ther 2000;80:128–140

33. Schlegel TF, Burks RT, Marcus RL, Dunn HK. A prospective evaluation of untreated acute grade III acromioclavicular separations. Am J Sports Med 2001;29: 699–703

34. Moseley JB Jr, Jobe FW, Pink M, Perry J, Tibone J. EMG analysis of the scapular muscles during a shoulder rehabilitation program. Am J Sports Med 1992;20: 128–134

35. Blackburn TA, McLoad WD, White B, Wofford L. EMG analysis of posterior rotator cuff exercises. Athletic Training 1990;25:40–45

36. Tibone J, Sellers R, Tonino P. Strength testing after third-degree acromioclavicular dislocations. Am J Sports Med 1992;20:328–331

37. Cordasco FA, Wolfe IN, Wootten ME, Bigliani LU. An electromyographic analysis of the shoulder during a medicine ball rehabilitation program. Am J Sports Med 1996;24:386–392

38. Davies GJ. A Compendium of Isokinetics in Clinical Usage and Rehabilitation Techniques. 4th ed. Onalaska, WI: S & S Publishing; 1992

# 6

# Classification and Treatment of Scapular Pathology

W. Ben Kibler

Scapular position and motion are closely integrated with arm motion to accomplish all shoulder functions. This integrated motion is called *scapulohumeral rhythm* (SHR). SHR is frequently altered in patients with shoulder injuries. Scapular dyskinesis, defined as alterations in normal resting scapular position or normal dynamic scapular motion, can affect many aspects of normal shoulder function, including the magnitude of the acromiohumeral distance in the subacromial space, the relation between the glenoid and the long axis of the humerus [the glenohumeral (GH) angle], the amount of posterior shoulder impingement, and the maximum possible activation of the rotator cuff muscles. These alterations may cause or increase the clinical manifestations of shoulder injury.

Scapular dyskinesis can be evaluated on physical exam; its treatment may be one of the keys to the treatment and rehabilitation of shoulder injury. In this chapter, normal SHR in shoulder function and abnormal rhythm in shoulder injury are reviewed, and guidelines are provided for shoulder evaluation and treatment.

## ◆ Scapulohumeral Rhythm in Shoulder Function

Many studies have evaluated scapular and arm motion and have reported on the coupled motions. These reports studied two-dimensional (2D) motion of arm elevation and scapular upward rotation.[1,2] They showed a composite humerus to scapular (H:S) ratio of 2:1, although the H:S ratio varied widely within segments of the arc of motion.

Recent work has examined scapular motion in a three-dimensional (3D) context. These studies have shown that scapular motion is a composite of three motions: (1) upward–downward rotation around a horizontal axis perpendicular to the plane of the scapula (**Fig. 6–1A**), (2) anterior–posterior tilt around a horizontal axis in the plane of the scapula (**Fig. 6–1B**), and (3) internal (IR) and external rotation (ER) around a vertical axis through the plane of the scapula (**Fig. 6–1C**).[3,4] There are two translations with an intact acromioclavicular (AC) joint:upward and downward translation on the thoracic wall and retraction–protraction around the ellipsoid

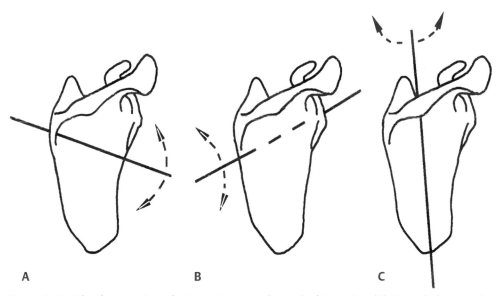

A               B               C

**Figure 6–1** The three motions that comprise normal scapular kinematics. **(A)** Upward–downward rotation around a horizontal axis perpendicular to the plane of the scapula. **(B)** Anterior–posterior tilt around a horizontal axis through the plane of the scapula. **(C)** External–internal rotation around a vertical axis through the plane of the scapula.

curve of the rib cage. In this more complex framework, the scapula is shown to have several roles in shoulder function. In addition to upward rotation, the scapula must also posteriorly tilt and externally rotate to clear the acromion from the moving arm.[3-5] Also, the scapula must internally and externally rotate and posteriorly tilt to maintain the glenoid as a congruent socket for the moving arm and maximize concavity and compression.[6] Finally, the scapula must be stabilized in a position of relative retraction during arm use to maximize activation of all the muscles that originate on the scapula.[7]

These positions and motions are produced and maintained by coordinated patterns of muscle activation that are preprogrammed and task specific.[1,8,9] They create force couples to stabilize and move the scapula and move the arm.[8,10,11] A predominant force couple pattern involves upper trapezius and serratus anterior activation to initiate scapular upward and ER, followed by lower trapezius activation to stabilize the rotated scapula and add additional posterior tilt as the arm is maximally elevated.[8] These activations precede maximal rotator cuff activation, allowing the cuff to contract off a stabilized base.[11] Another important force couple includes middle trapezius: serratus anterior working as external rotators of the scapula. Finally, the lower trapezius is coupled with the latissimus dorsi to rotate the elevated arm on the stabilized scapula.

## ◆ Scapular Dysfunction in Shoulder Injury

Scapular dyskinesis is found in a high percentage of patients with shoulder injuries.[4,5,10,12] Biomechanical studies reveal that the dyskinesis is a combination of decreased posterior tilt and decreased ER as well as decreased upward rotation.[4,5] Clinical studies on dyskinesis have been difficult because of the inability to "see" the scapula because of the multiple possible positions and the muscular covering. The predominant finding on clinical exam is a prominence of the medial border of the scapula upon observation at rest or upon motion of the arm in elevation. This finding has been broken down into the most common patterns that are observed. The most common patterns include inferior border prominence (type I), entire medial border prominence (type II), or superior medial border prominence (type III) (**Fig. 6–2**).[13] These patterns are consistent with the three possible motions in 3D space. The patterns may occur singly in one patient, but they commonly occur in combinations of patterns as the arms move. They are not specifically associated with any particular shoulder injuries, but types I and II are more commonly seen with instabilities and labral injuries, and types I and III are more commonly associated with rotator cuff injuries.

These patterns represent loss of dynamic control of the translation of scapular retraction and the motion of ER. Scapular retraction is regarded as a key element in closed chain coupled SHR.[1,3,4] If this control is lost, gravity, forward arm motion, and muscle activations take the arm and shoulder girdle forward. The biomechanical result is a tendency toward scapular IR and protraction around the rib cage. Excessive scapular protraction alters the scapular roles in shoulder function.[14] The normal timing and magnitude of acromial motion are changed, the subacromial space distance is altered, the GH arm angle may be increased, producing the "hyperangulated" joint, and maximal muscle activation may be decreased. These patterns appear to be independent from the various diagnoses of shoulder injury, such as AC joint arthrosis, GH internal derangement or instability, biceps tendinopathy, or labral injury. They appear to be the result of abnormal muscle activations, either directly due to muscle involvement or to neurologically based inhibition, or alteration in muscle activation patterns from a wide variety of causative factors.

Causative factors for scapular dyskinesis may be broadly classified into proximal (to the scapula) and distal types.[15] Proximal causative factors are most frequently because of direct alteration of muscle properties, such as inflexibility, weakness, fatigue, or nerve injury, and are usually treated by rehabilitation. Muscle weakness has been demonstrated in the serratus anterior[5,16] and lower trapezius[5] in impingement patients. This has been shown to be due to fatigue and inhibition of activation.[16] Occasionally, it will be the result of a direct injury due to trauma. Alteration in muscle

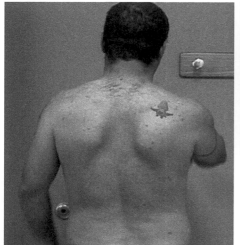

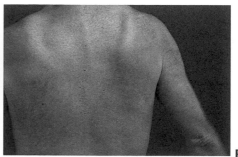

**B**

**A**

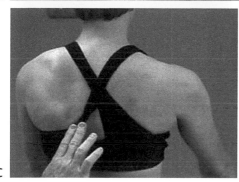

**C**

**Figure 6–2** Patterns of scapular dyskinesis. **(A)** Inferior medial border prominence. **(B)** Medial border prominence. **(C)** Superior medial border prominence.

activation patterns, with delayed upper trapezius activation, has also been demonstrated.[10] Inflexibility in the pectoralis minor is a common finding in impingement. This has been shown to be an absolute decrease in muscle length and an increased muscle activation in response to tensile loads.[17] A relatively rare proximal cause is true nerve injury to the long thoracic or accessory nerve. Bony proximal causes include thoracic kyphosis or scoliosis, with resultant alteration in scapular position. A surgically treatable proximal cause is lower or middle trapezius muscle detachment off the medial border, either due to trauma or because of surgical treatment of snapping scapula syndrome. Traumatic detachment is rare but has been seen after tensile stretch over a seat belt in vehicular accidents or after direct blows. If a patient has the same or worse symptoms

after snapping scapula surgery, the muscles may not be properly attached.

Distal causative factors are most commonly due to anatomic injuries in the AC or GH joints. They also alter muscle activation patterns or activations by causing instability of the bones or through pain-based inhibition, but frequently require surgical treatment to eliminate their effects and provide the basis for effective rehabilitation. GH instability is associated with altered serratus anterior activation[18]; GH instability and rotator cuff injury are associated with altered SHR that improves after surgical treatment.[19] Superior glenoid labral tears are associated with dyskinesis in 94% of the cases.[20]

A common distal causative factor that rarely needs surgical treatment is glenohumeral internal rotation deficit (GIRD). GIRD is defined as side-to-side asymmetry of >25

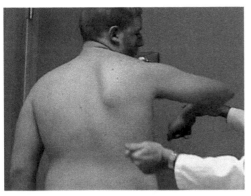

**Figure 6–3** "Wind-up" of the scapula on the flexed arm due to tight posterior capsule and shortened muscles. To complete the forward motion, the scapula must protract around the ribs.

degrees or an absolute value of <25 degrees.[20] It is thought to be produced by acquired posterior capsular contracture and posterior muscle stiffness and is frequently seen in all types of shoulder injuries.[20,21] GIRD creates abnormal scapular kinematics because of the "wind up" effect of the arm on the scapula. As the arm is forward flexed, horizontally adducted, and internally rotated in throwing or working, the tight capsule and muscles pull the scapula into a protracted, internally rotated and anteriorly tilted position, which causes downward rotation of the acromion (**Fig. 6–3**).

Scapular dyskinesis can affect the clinical presentation of both classical or external impingement and internal impingement. In external impingement because of decreased posterior tilt and upward rotation, the dyskinetic position causes the acromion to not elevate, placing increased pressure on the rotator cuff and subacromial space with arm elevation.[4,5] In internal impingement, the dyskinetic position because of excessive scapular internal rotation and protraction creates glenoid antetilting with increased mechanical abutment of the humerus and supraspinatus against the glenoid and labrum, creating labral tears and the "dead arm" syndrome.[20] The dyskinetic position of protraction also increases tensile load on the anterior band of the inferior GH ligament, creating a stretched ligament that is more likely to allow anterior translation[20,22]

## ◆ Physical Examination of the Scapula in Shoulder Injury

In a physical exam of the scapula, the goals are to establish the presence or absence of scapular dyskinesis, to evaluate proximal and distal causative factors, and to employ dynamic maneuvers to assess the effect of correction of dyskinesis on impingement symptoms. The results of the exam will aid in establishing the complete diagnosis of all the elements of the dysfunction and will help guide treatment and rehabilitation.

The scapular exam should largely be accomplished from the posterior aspect.[6] The scapula should be exposed for complete visualization. You may ask the patient to don a gown. Or simply have the male patient remove his shirt; a woman may be advised prior to the appointment to wear a tank top or a sports bra to the exam. The resting posture should be checked for side-to-side asymmetry but especially for evidence of inferior medial or medial border prominence (**Fig. 6–2**). If there is difficulty with determining the positions, marking the superior and inferior medial borders may help to ascertain the position.

Dynamic scapular motions may be evaluated by having the patient move the arms in ascent and descent three to five times. This will usually bring out any weakness in the muscles and display the dyskinetic patterns. If necessary, more repetitions, up to 10, or addition of 3- to 5-lb weights will highlight the weakness even more. Alteration in medial scapular border motion in any plane, singly or in combination, is recorded in a "yes" (present) or "no" (absent) fashion. This evaluation system allows a higher degree of reliability between the clinical exam and the biomechanical findings. Evaluation based on the single patterns had only a 0.49 to 0.54 correlation with biomechanical findings.[13] The clinically observed "yes/no" evaluation had a 0.84 correlation with biomechanically determined abnormalities in symptomatic patients; thus, it has a high predictive value.[23]

Corrective maneuvers that may alter the injury symptoms are important to give information about the role of scapular dyskinesis in the total picture of dysfunction that accompanies shoulder injury and needs to be restored.

In this regard, the scapular assistance test (SAT) and the scapular retraction test (SRT) are useful. In the SAT (**Fig. 6–4**), the examiner applies gentle pressure to assist scapular upward rotation and posterior tilt as the patient elevates the arm. A positive result occurs when the painful arc impingement symptoms are relieved and the arc of motion is increased. In the SRT (**Fig. 6–5**), the examiner places and stabilizes the scapula in a retracted position. There are two possible positive results. The first occurs when the demonstrated supraspinatus strength, determined by manual muscle testing, is increased in the retracted position. The second occurs when symptoms of internal impingement and posterior superior labral injury, determined by the ER relocation maneuver or the Mayo shear test, are diminished or relieved by retraction. A positive SAT or SRT shows that scapular dyskinesis is directly involved in producing the symptoms and indicates the need for inclusion of early scapular rehabilitation exercises to improve scapular control.

The lateral scapular slide (LSS) (**Fig. 6–6**) is a semidynamic measurement of scapular control. To determine the bilateral measurements of the distance between the inferior medial scapular tip and the spine, the arms are in 80 to 90 degrees of abduction and maximally internally rotated. In this modified LSS, measuring only one arm position, side-to-side asymmetries of >1.5 cm have a 0.84 correlation with biomechanically determined excessive scapular IR.[24]

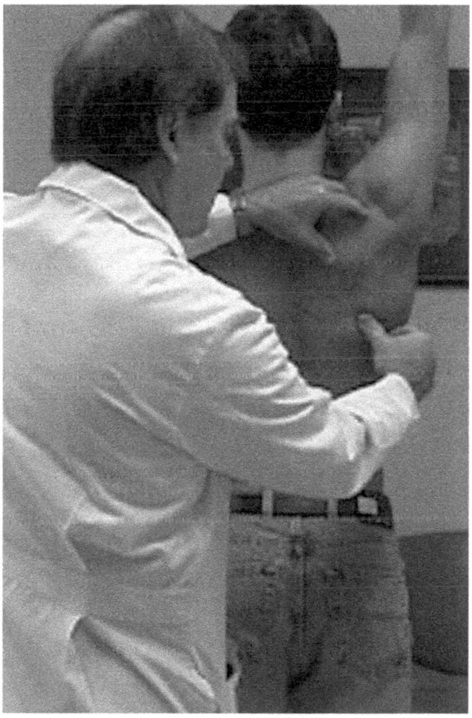

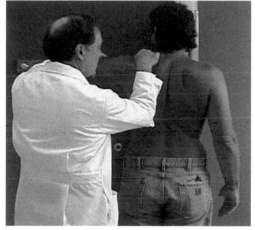

**Figure 6–5** The scapular retraction test (SRT). The examiner stabilizes the scapula in a retracted position and rechecks manual muscle strength or posterior impingement symptoms.

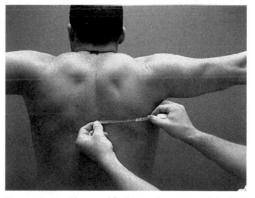

**Figure 6–6** The modified lateral scapular slide (LSS). The measurement is from the inferior scapula tip to the nearest spinous process.

**Figure 6–4** The scapular assistance test (SAT). The examiner dynamically assists upward rotation and posterior tilt as the patient elevates the arm. Minimal pressure is exerted.

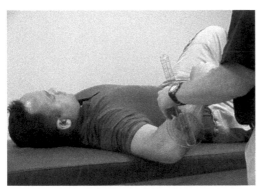

**Figure 6–7** Glenohumeral (GH) internal rotation measured from a stabilized scapula with a goniometer. Rotation should be taken to tightness in the GH motion or until the scapula winds up off the table.

Evaluation of GIRD should be done by stabilizing the scapula, placing the arm in 90 degrees of abduction in the scapular plane, and rotating the arm (**Fig. 6–7**). Rotation should be taken to tightness in the motion and/or when the scapula starts to move forward in a wind-up fashion. Bilateral measurements should be obtained. GIRD does not correlate with the spinous-level method of estimating shoulder IR because there are at least 7 degrees of freedom in the spinous-level measurement test, only one of which is GH internal rotation.[25] Because GH internal rotation is the abnormal biomechanical motion, it should be tested specifically.

Coracoid-based inflexibility can be assessed by palpation of the pectoralis minor and the biceps short head as they run off the coracoid tip. They will usually be tender to palpation, even if they are not symptomatic in use, can be traced to their insertions as taut bands, and will create symptoms of soreness and stiffness when the scapula are manually maximally retracted. A rough measurement of pectoralis minor tightness can be obtained by standing the patient against the wall and measuring the distance from the wall to the anterior acromial tip.

Proximal factors influencing scapular dyskinesis may be evaluated in a screening fashion. Hip/trunk stability can be assessed by the single-leg stability series, which consists of single-leg stance and single-leg squat maneuvers (**Fig. 6–8**).[6] Trunk flexibility may be evaluated by standard sit and reach and lateral bending exercises. Periscapular muscle strength weakness can be assessed by watching scapular position for dyskinesis during wall pushups. Isolated serratus anterior and trapezius can be done for nerve-related palsies. Any deficits found on the screening exam should be evaluated in more depth. It is common to find some evidence of proximal muscle weakness or inflexibility, which will affect the optimum mechanics of SHR. This may not be the sole factor but must be included in the rehabilitation protocols.[26]

Distal factors influencing scapular dyskinesis may be assessed by standard physical exam techniques for GH and AC joint internal derangements. Tests should include evaluation of rotator cuff strength and integrity, GH instability, superior labral tears, biceps tendinopathy, and AC joint arthrosis or instability.

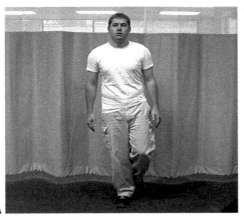
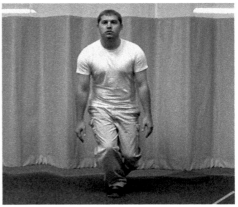

**Figure 6–8** Single-leg stability series. **(A)** Single-leg stance. Watch for Trendelenberg posture. **(B)** Single-leg squat. Squat to 45 degrees. Watch for rotation or trunk lean.

## ◆ Treatment Guidelines

Treatment of scapular dyskinesis should proceed along two pathways: appropriately addressing any proximal or distal causative factors that require surgery, and reestablishing normal scapular kinematics through physical therapy.[26,27]

Surgical treatment would address any muscle detachments from the scapula, any GH internal derangement or instability, rotator cuff partial or complete tears, biceps/rotator interval injury, or AC joint injury. For both the surgical repair and the scapular dyskinesis, the patient would undergo rehabilitation.

Rehabilitation of scapular dyskinesis should start with restoration of flexibility. "Sleeper" stretches (**Fig. 6–9**) are excellent for improving GIRD, and "open book" stretches (**Fig. 6–10**) can improve coracoid-based inflexibility. General flexibility exercises for the trunk should also be included. As muscle rehabilitation is started, the patient should continue the flexibility exercises.

Muscle strength in the periscapular muscles is often very weak in patients with long-standing shoulder injury; this is due to disuse and inhibition. Early strengthening should not be done by isolating these weak muscles. The early exercises should take advantage of the facilitation of the periscapular activation by the synergistic proximal trunk and hip muscle activations. They also will allow proximal kinetic chain activation. Because these exercises are done in a closed chain fashion, they also do not put excessive loads on the impinged or injured distal structures.[27] Exercise sets should include integrated hip extension/trunk extension/scapular retractions (lawn mower pulls) close to, then farther away from the body (**Fig. 6–11**); scapular pinches, integrated trunk extension/scapular

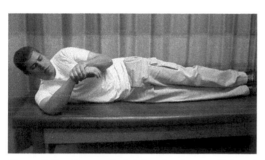

**Figure 6–9** Sleeper stretch for glenohumeral internal rotation deficit (GIRD). Stabilize the scapula and rotate the arm to tightness.

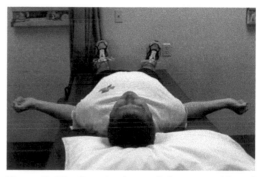

**Figure 6–10** Open book stretch for coracoid-based tightness. Keep arms <90 degrees abduction to decrease thoracic outlet symptoms.

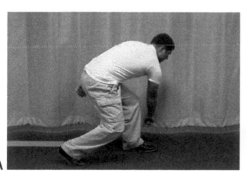

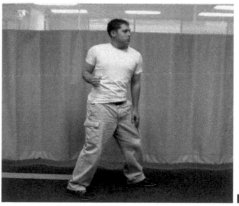

A      B

**Figure 6–11** Lawn mower pulls. Start with the arm close to the body **(A),** then move the arm away to get more scapular control **(B)**. May be done in ipsilateral or diagonal patterns.

retraction/arm extension (low rows) (**Fig. 6–12**); and closed chain scapular clock exercises (**Fig. 6–13**).[26,27] All the exercises start and end in the "ideal position" of trunk extension and scapular retraction. Because these muscles are often inhibited and the normal activation patterns are not present, many verbal, tactile, and visual clues are necessary in the early stages of rehabilitation. Some common verbal cues include "lift your sternum," "stand up straight," "put your elbows in your back pockets," and "cock your shoulders." Tactile cues include taping, pressure on the lower trapezius, and various proprioceptive braces that are being developed. Visual cues include standing in front of a mirror and making sure the shoulders are at the same height, standing between two mirrors so the patient can see the scapular posture, and the "doorway reminder"—every time the patient walks through a doorway, put "elbows in their back pockets."

Rotator cuff activation is key to humeral head depression and GH concavity and compression. Shoulder function is maximized by maximal rotator cuff activation. Maximal rotator cuff activation only occurs on the base of a stabilized scapula, and in force couple activation. Rotator cuff emphasis in the rehabilitation of most shoulder injuries should be later in the flow of the rehabilitation protocol, after establishment of proximal stability, and should emphasize cocontraction of the muscles in force couples and integrated scapular stabilization/humeral head depression exercises (**Fig. 6–14**). A study has shown that different types of exercises place different loads on the rotator cuff.[28] Based on this study, progression in rotator cuff exercises should be from closed to open chain position, from horizontal to vertical to diagonal direction, and from slow to fast speed. Each type of progression increases rotator cuff muscle activation.[28]

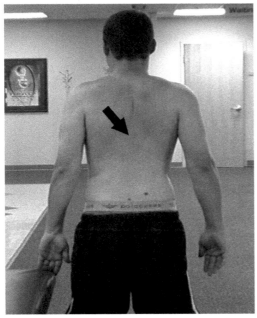

**Figure 6–12** Low row. This is an excellent exercise to start early in rehabilitation. The arm is safely at the side to decrease impingement symptoms and positions. The patient retracts and depresses the scapula (direction of arrow).

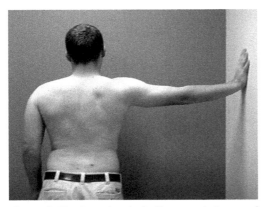

**Figure 6–13** Scapular clock. The scapula is moved into different clock positions with the arm at different elevations. The closed chain position decreases the load on the arm and decreases impingement symptoms.

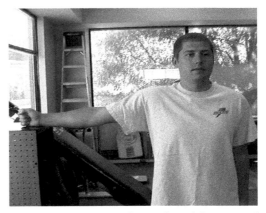

**Figure 6–14** Integrated scapula stabilization and humeral head depression. This allows rotator cuff activation in patterns to replicate rotator cuff function.

## ◆ Summary

Scapular dyskinesis is frequently associated with the clinical presentation of patients with shoulder injury due to the alteration of the obligatory biomechanical coupling of scapular and arm motion, which occurs in normal shoulder function and is lost when patients develop symptoms. Clinical evaluation of the scapula should be a normal part of the evaluation of patients with external or internal impingement, rotator cuff injury, labral tears, or GH instability. The treatment and rehabilitation of a shoulder injury should include the scapula when dyskinesis is demonstrated.

# References

1. Happee R, van der Helm FC. The control of shoulder muscles during goal directed movements: an inverse dynamic analysis. J Biomech 1995;28:1179–1191

2. Bagg SD, Forrest WJ. A biomechanical analysis of scapular rotations during arm rotation abduction in the scapular plane. Am J Phys Med Rehabil 1988; 67:238–245

3. McClure PW, Michener LA, Sennett BJ, Karduna AR. Direct 3-dimensional measurement of scapular kinematics during dynamic movements in vivo. J Shoulder Elbow Surg 2001;10:269–277

4. Lukasiewicz AC, McClure PW, Michener LA, Pratt N, Sennett B. Comparison of 3-dimensional scapular positions and orientation between subjects with and without shoulder impingement. J Orthop Sports Phys Ther 1999;29:574–586

5. Ludewig PM, Cook TM. Alterations in shoulder kinematics and associated muscle activity in people with symptoms of shoulder impingement. Phys Ther 2000;80:276–291

6. Kibler WB, McMullen J. Scapular dyskinesis and its relation to shoulder pain. J Am Acad Orthop Surg 2003;11:142–152

7. Kebatse M, McClure PW, Pratt N. Thoracic position effect on shoulder range of motion, strength, and 3-dimensional scapular kinematics. Arch Phys Med Rehab 1999;80:945–950

8. Bagg SD, Forrest WJ. Electromyographic study of the scapular rotators during arm abduction in the scapular plane. Am J Phys Med 1986;65:111–124

9. Prilutsky BI, Zatsiorsky VM. Optimization based models of muscle coordination. Exerc Sports Sci Rev 2002; 30:32–38

10. Cools A, Witvrouw E, DeClercq G, Danneels LA, Cambier DC. Scapular muscle recruitment pattern: trapezius muscle latency in overhead athletes with and without impingement symptoms. Am J Sports Med 2003;31:542–549

11. Speer K, Garrett WE. Muscular control of motion and stability about the pectoral girdle. In: Matsen FA, Fu F,

Hawkins RJ, eds. The Shoulder: A Balance of Mobility and Stability. Rosemont IL: AAOS; 1993:159–172

12. Warner JP, Micheli LJ, Arslanian LE, et al. Scapulohumeral motion in normal shoulders and in shoulders with instability and impingement syndrome. Clin Orthop Relat Res 1991;285:191–199

13. Kibler WB, Uhl TL, Maddux JW, et al. Qualitative clinical evaluation of scapular dysfunction: a reliability study. J Shoulder Elbow Surg 2002;11:550–556

14. Kibler WB. The role of the scapula in athletic shoulder function. Am J Sports Med 1998;26:325–337

15. Rubin B, Kibler WB. Fundamental principles of shoulder rehabilitation: conservative to postoperative management. Arthroscopy 2002;18(Suppl):29–39

16. Cools A, Witvrouw E, DeClercq G, Vanderstraeten GG, Cambier DC. Evaluation of isokinetic force production and associated muscle activity in the scapular rotators during a retraction-protraction movement in overhead athletes with impingement symptoms. Br J Sports Med 2004;38:64–68

17. Borstad JD, Ludewig PM. The effect of long versus short pectoralis minor resting lengths on scapular kinematics. J Orthop Sports Phys Ther 2005;35: 227–238

18. Glousman R, Jobe F, Tibone J, et al. Dynamic electromyographic analysis of the throwing shoulder with glenohumeral instability. J Bone Joint Surg Am 1988;70A:220–226

19. Paletta GA, Warner JJP, Warren RF, et al. Shoulder kinematics with 2 plane x-ray evaluation in patients with anterior instability or rotator cuff tears. J Shoulder Elbow Surg 1997;6:516–527

20. Burkhart SS, Morgan CD, Kibler WB. Current concepts: the disabled throwing shoulder: spectrum of pathology, I: Pathoanatomy and biomechanics. Arthroscopy 2003;19:404–420

21. Tyler TF, Nicholas SJ, Roy T, et al. Quantification of posterior capsule tightness and motion loss in patients with shoulder impingement. Am J Sports Med 2000;28:668–673

22. Weiser WM, Lee TQ, McMaster WC. Effects of simulated scapular protraction on anterior glenohumeral stability. Am J Sports Med 1999;27:801–805

23. Kibler WB, Tripp BL, Uhl TL. 3-dimensional scapular kinematics in injured and noninjured subjects: relation to clinical observation of scapular dyskinesis. J Shoulder Elbow Surg 2005

24. Schwellnus MP. The repeatability of clinical and laboratory tests to measure scapular position and movement during arm abduction. Intl Sports Med J 2003; 4:1–10

25. Mallon WJ, Herring CL, Sallay PI, et al. Use of vertebral levels to measure presumed internal rotation at the shoulder: a radiographic analysis. J Shoulder Elbow Surg 1996;5:299–306

26. McMullen J, Uhl TL. A kinetic chain approach for shoulder rehabilitation. J Ath Training 2000;35: 329–337

27. Kibler WB, Livingston BP. Closed chain rehabilitation for upper and lower extremities. J Am Acad Orthop Surg 2001;9:412–423

28. Wise MB, Uhl TL, Mattacola AJ, Nitz AJ, Kibler WB. The effect of limb support on muscle activation during shoulder exercises. J Shoulder Elbow Surg 2004; 13:614–620

# II

# Special Topics in Shoulder Rehabilitation

# 7

# Modification of Traditional Exercises for Shoulder Rehabilitation and a Return-to-Lifting Program

**Jake Bleacher and Todd S. Ellenbecker**

Traditional upper-body weightlifting exercises such as the bench press, military press, and latissimus dorsi (lat) pull-downs are just a few of the regularly performed resistance exercises included in many training programs utilized by the recreational weightlifter, bodybuilder, or competitive athlete to enhance strength, performance, body composition, and aesthetics. The unique anatomy and biomechanics of the shoulder girdle present an increased risk of injury with many of the traditional weightlifting exercises, which exceed the mobility and stability requirements of the shoulder complex.[1] Although many of these exercises are recognized by physical therapists and athletic trainers as inappropriate during shoulder rehabilitation, many patients hope to return to performing these exercises at some point following their recovery from shoulder injury or surgery. Furthermore, high resistance, low-repetition formats using traditional weightlifting exercises are not a recommended component of rehabilitation programs but do form the mainstay of many strength and conditioning programs for athletes.[2] During rehabilitation of the shoulder following injury or surgery, patients whose primary recreational activity involves traditional weightlifting at the local gym must be given some exercise guidance and parameters to prevent reinjury and allow a continued exercise program for general health and performance enhancement.

In this chapter, we will give an overview of the specific stresses on the human shoulder inherent in many traditional weightlifting exercises and provide modifications to these exercises to protect the static and dynamic stabilizing structures. We will also outline specific strategies and concepts for patients following shoulder injury and/or surgical procedures such as rotator cuff tendonitis, acromioclavicular (AC) joint pathology, glenohumeral (GH) joint instability, and labral repair.

## ◆ Stresses on the Shoulder of Traditional Upper-Extremity Resistive Exercise

Although many stresses are indeed present during the performance of upper-extremity resisted exercise, we will focus on the impingement stresses inherent in exercises using overhead positioning, as well as the tensile loading to the GH joint capsular ligaments during performance of movements or exercises behind the scapular and coronal planes of the body.

The stresses inherent in traditional weightlifting exercise can exaggerate the compressive forces against the undersurface of the acromion outlined by Wuelker et al.[3] Many traditional exercises such as the lateral raise, triceps pullover, and military press utilize ranges of motion (ROM) with greater than 90 degrees of elevation. Wuelker et al[3] found that peak subacromial forces occur between 85 and 120 degrees, with peak forces estimated at 0.42 times body weight or 10.2 times the weight of the upper extremity in unloaded conditions.[4] These stresses are magnified in the presence of subacromial spurs, AC injury, and acromial types II and III, which increase the incidence of rotator cuff tears[5,6] and can be present in the skeletally mature weightlifter presenting with shoulder pain.

Additionally, many traditional resistance exercises used by weightlifters and body builders place large stresses on the anterior glenohumeral ligament complex.[1,7] The anterior band of the inferior glenohumeral ligament is an important structure responsible for stabilizing against anterior, posterior, and inferior GH translation with 90 degrees of GH abduction.[7] The stresses on this structure are increased during exercise movements that place the shoulder behind the coronal plane of the body (**Fig. 7–1**) such as the end-range descent phase of the bench press, the pushup, the pec deck, as well as during the behind-the-head lat pull-down, and during exercises such as the dip and behind-the-head overhead shoulder press. Fees et al[2] have termed the abduction external rotation (ER) position inherent in many of these aforementioned exercises as the *high-five position* and have recommended modifications to this position for patients returning to traditional weightlifting programs following injury or surgery as well as for high-risk groups, which include overhead athletes and those with underlying GH joint hypermobility.

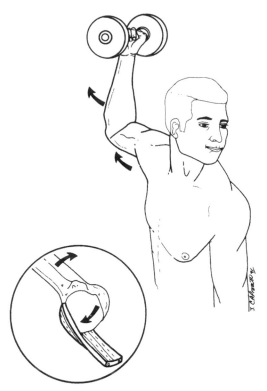

**Figure 7–1** The at-risk position or high-five position. Inset shows the stress on the anterior band of the inferior glenohumeral joint ligament. (From Gross ML, Brenner S, Esformes I, Sonzogni JJ. Anterior shoulder instability in weight lifters. Am J Sports Medicine1993; 21:601, **Fig. 2.** Reprinted by permission.)

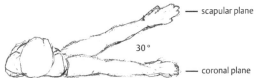

**Figure 7–2** Glenohumeral joint abduction in the scapular and coronal planes. (Figure 7–2 courtesy of Veronica Serna.)

## Anatomic and Biomechanical Rationale for Range-of-Motion Limitation in Traditional Upper-Extremity Resistive Exercise

Many of the traditional overhead pushing and pulling lifts (military press, pull-downs, chin-ups, deltoid laterals) cause an increased stress to the inferior and anterior portion of the GH capsule and ligaments, along with an increased risk of subacromial impingement. Overhead lifting movements that position the shoulder in end-range abduction increase the stress to the static stabilizers of the shoulder, while at the same time decreasing the mechanical efficiency of the dynamic stabilizers of the shoulder girdle.[8] The mechanical disadvantage in these end-range overhead positions is because of a decrease in the anatomic length–tension relationship of the shoulder abductors and rotators with the scapular stabilizers. This less-than-optimal relationship between the dynamic stabilizing muscles of the shoulder and scapular muscles places increased demands on the static and dynamic stabilizers, and attenuation of these structures should stability requirements not be met.[9] The scapular plane position, which is 30 to 45 degrees anterior to the coronal plane, reorients the humerus and scapula to a more advantageous position (**Fig. 7–2**).[10] The scapular plane position of the shoulder reduces the capsuloligamentous stress and creates an optimal anatomic length–tension relationship for the scapular and rotator cuff muscles.[11]

## General Strategies to Protect the Shoulder during Weightlifting Exercises

There is a greater risk for injuries to the shoulder than in other large synovial joints such as the hip and knee because of the inherent instability of the GH joint, which is characterized by incongruity of the articulating surfaces and lack of osseous stability.[8]

Coupled with the excessive range of motion afforded to the shoulder complex, there exists a vulnerability to the static and dynamic restraints in the shoulder when the arm is loaded with resistance beyond optimal anatomic safe zones. The *safe zone*, as identified by the second author[9] in the development of an upper-extremity tennis conditioning program, consists of performing resistive exercises below shoulder level (90 degrees of shoulder elevation) and anterior to the coronal plane (optimally the scapular plane) to minimize subacromial impingement and prevent abnormal stress to the anterior GH joint capsule and capsular ligaments (**Fig. 7–3**).[2] In the remainder of this chapter, we will identify traditional weightlifting exercises that are

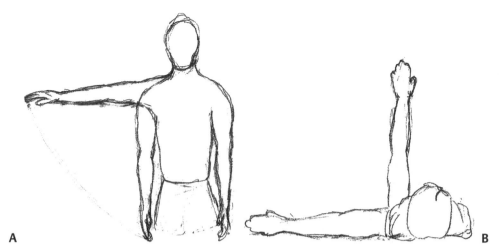

A                                                                          B

**Figure 7–3**  Safe-zone general guideline depicting range of motion limitation for modification of traditional weightlifting exercises. (Figure 7–3 courtesy of Veronica Serna.)

potentially harmful to a patient recovering from a shoulder injury, and suggest modifications to traditional exercise(s) to gain the benefit of stressing the targeted muscle without placing undue strain on the stabilizing structures of the shoulder. Specific recommendations are given for each exercise along with detailed photos to facilitate the proper application of the exercise modifications.

It is assumed that the patient or individual for whom these exercises are intended has reached a level of recovery and function, particularly acceptable levels of rotator cuff and scapular strength, endurance, and optimal external–internal rotation balance and force couple relationships. The treating physician or the appropriate rehabilitation personnel should discuss with the patient and approve any resumption of an exercise program, particularly weightlifting or sports activities.

### Specific Concepts for Modification of Weightlifting Exercises

Before individually covering specific weightlifting exercises and movement patterns, we will review several concepts in relation to grip position and hand placement that apply to many traditional weightlifting exercises.

In addition to maintaining the shoulder in a position near the scapular plane, other components of a lift, such as the hand spacing

and grip type (overhand, underhand, and neutral rotation) can be modified to decrease shoulder torque and tendon impingement. In general, hand placement is typically gauged relative to the width between the lifter's acromion process. Wider hand spacing (>1.5 × shoulder or biacromial distance) (**Fig. 7–4**) for traditional lifts such as the flat, incline, and decline bench press, military press, barbell squats, and pull-downs are generally not recommended in patients with either anterior shoulder instability or subacromial impingement and rotator cuff pathology because of the increased stability requirements and torque generated at the shoulder.[2,12] When the rotator cuff is either compromised or has insufficient strength, there is a greater likelihood of GH instability when greater demands are placed on the dynamic stabilizers and they are not met. To minimize this stress, hand spacing should be no greater than 1.5 × the biacromial width, unless there is evidence of posterior shoulder instability. In patients with posterior instability, it is generally recommended to utilize wider hand spacing to limit the stress on the posterior restraints (hand spacing greater than 1.5 × the biacromial width) (**Fig. 7–5**). The wider hand spacing allows for better approximation of the humeral head in the glenoid fossa.[2]

The actual grip type will also affect subacromial spacing for the supraspinatus and long

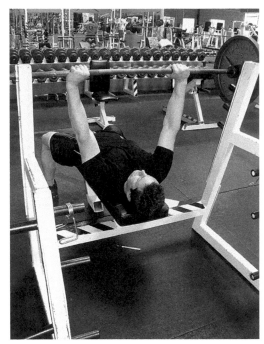

**Figure 7–4** Bench press exercise with hand spacing 1.5 × the biacromial width. This position is recommended for individuals with a history of rotator cuff pathology and anterior glenohumeral joint instability.

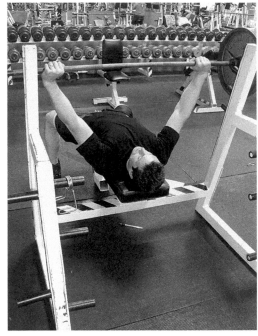

**Figure 7–5** Bench press exercise with hand spacing >1.5 × the biacromial width. This hand position would be recommended for individuals with a history of posterior glenohumeral joint instability.

head of the biceps tendon. Consideration of the type of pathology present will affect grip selection. The overhand (fully pronated forearm) grip (**Fig. 7–6**) will remove the long head of the biceps from below the acromion because of the internally rotated position of the humerus, but at the same time will draw the supraspinatus tendon under the acromion.[2] This overhand position can cause tethering of the supraspinatus tendon if a hooked acromion or primary impingement is present. Using the overhand grip will place the biceps tendon in a position where it will be less likely to be contacted under the acromion.[13,14] The underhand grip (fully supinated forearm) (**Fig. 7–7**) allows the supraspinatus to be drawn outside of the subacromial space, but at the same time brings the tendinous portion of the long head of the biceps tendon under the acromion; this may cause impingement of the long head of the biceps tendon.[2] A neutral hand positioning (forearms resting in neutral pronation and supination) allows for a more anatomically optimal relationship for the tendinous attachments to the anterolateral humeral head

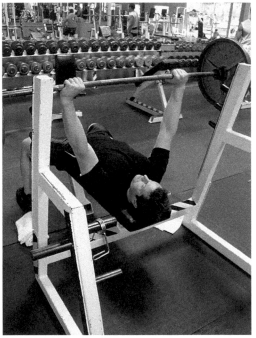

**Figure 7–6** Bench press with traditional overhand or pronated grip.

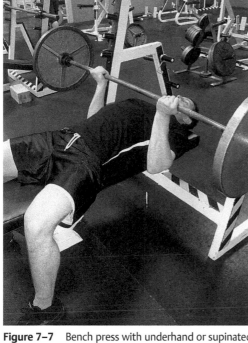

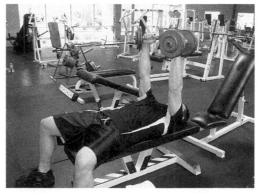

**Figure 7–8** Photo of dumbbell bench press with neutral forearm grip.

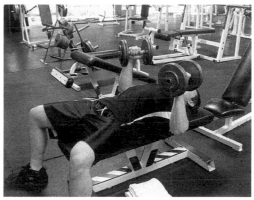

**Figure 7–9** Photo of dumbbell shoulder press with neutral forearm grip.

**Figure 7–7** Bench press with underhand or supinated grip.

when the arm spacing is shoulder-width apart. This neutral forearm position is possible with dumbbells (**Figs. 7–8 and 7–9**) or on weight machines designed with variable grip types. Additional grip modifications are pictured in **Figures 7–10 and 7–11** for the seated row and lat pull-down, respectively.

### ◆ Modifications of Specific Weightlifting Exercises

**Tables 7–1** to **7–5** provide summaries of the recommended modifications of traditional weightlifting exercises, which are based on the anatomic and biomechanical concepts discussed in this chapter. They provide the clinician or therapist with an objective guide to returning a patient to traditional weightlifting exercises.

#### The Bench Press

The bench press, of all the chest exercises is one of the most widely used for developing and measuring upper-body strength and performance.[15] Because of the importance of the bench press exercise to weightlifters and many athletes, modifications to various elements of the exercise are necessary for those who are recovering from shoulder injury or surgery. Modifications to resistance, hand spacing, grip selection, and ROM in the GH joint are needed to minimize excess strain to the static and dynamic structures of the shoulder (**Table 7–1**). Early focus should be on adhering to correct form with lighter resistance and higher repetitions (12 to 15 RM loads). As mentioned in a previous section, hand spacing should be slightly wider than shoulder width apart (1 to 1.5 × biacromial width) with grip type (overhand, underhand, and neutral) varied based on the type of underlying pathology.

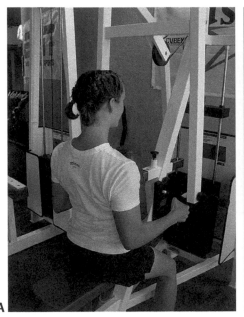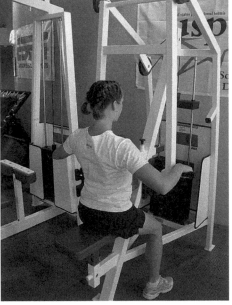

A

B

**Figure 7–10** Machine seated row with option of variable grip positions.

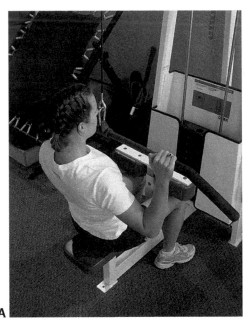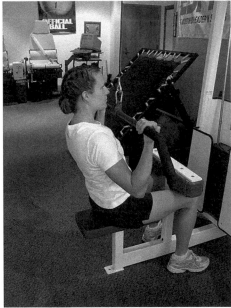

A

B

**Figure 7–11** Latissimus dorsi pull-down with **(A)** overhand and **(B)** underhand grip options.

Use of a narrow handgrip results in shoulder abduction angles limited to between 45 to 75 degrees, which minimizes the occurrence of subacromial impingement and AC joint compressive forces. Additionally, use of the narrow hand placement ($\leq 1.5 \times$ biacromial width) limits the amount of shoulder extension to less than 15 degrees. This minimizes the amount of horizontal abduction at the bottom of the lift, which is extremely important in reducing

**Table 7–1**   Modifications for Bench Press Exercises

| Exercise | Shoulder Pathology | Modifications |
|---|---|---|
| Flat bench press | Anterior instability | • Grip: <1.5 × biacromial width<br>• ROM limitations: <15 degrees shoulder extension (towel on chest, physioball, Smith machine spot blocks) |
| Flat bench press | Subacromial impingement | • Grip: narrow (1 to 1.5 × biacromial width), underhand grip<br>• ROM limitations: shoulder abduction between 45 to 75 degrees, shoulder extension <15 degrees |
| Flat bench press | SLAP lesion, long head of biceps pathology | • Grip: narrow (1 to 1.5 × biacromial width), overhand grip position<br>• ROM limitations: shoulder abduction between 45 to 75 degrees, shoulder extension <15 degrees |
| Flat bench press | AC joint pathology | • Grip: narrow (1 to 1.5 × biacromial width<br>• ROM limitations: shoulder abduction angles between 45 to 75 degrees, shoulder extension <15 degrees using towel on chest, Smith machine, physioball |
| Flat bench press | Posterior instability | • Grip: wide (>2 × biacromial width)<br>• ROM: 75 to 90 GH abduction |

AC, acromioclavicular; GH, glenohumeral, ROM, range of motion; SLAP, superior labrum anterior posterior.

**Table 7–2**   Modifications for Additional Chest Exercises

| Exercise | Shoulder Pathology | Modifications |
|---|---|---|
| Cable flies | Anterior instability, subacromial impingement | • Hand spacing: 1 to 1.5 × biacromial width<br>• ROM limitations: shoulder extension, horizontal abduction anterior to coronal plane<br>• GH abduction angles <90 degrees maintaining elbows below shoulder level |
| Pec deck | Anterior instability, subacromial impingement | • ROM limitations: shoulder horizontal abduction anterior to coronal plane<br>• GH abduction angles <90 degrees adjusting seat level |
| Dumbbell flies | Anterior instability, subacromial impingement, long head of biceps pathology | • ROM limitations: shoulder horizontal abduction, extension anterior to coronal plane (Swiss ball or wide bench limiting movement)<br>• GH abduction angles between 45 to 70 degrees<br>• Elbow flexion angles 70 to 90 degrees |
| Traditional pushup | Anterior instability, subacromial impingement, AC joint arthrosis | • Hand spacing: <1.5 × biacromial width<br>• ROM limitations: shoulder horizontal abduction anterior to coronal plane (medicine ball, at sternal level)<br>• GH abduction 15 to 70 degrees<br>• End-range plus position |

AC, acromioclavicular; GH, glenohumeral, ROM, range of motion.

anterior capsular stress and humeral head shear.[2] In addition to using a narrower grip, using a towel roll placed across the chest (**Fig. 7–12**), performing the lift within a Smith machine using spot blocks (**Fig. 7–13**), or by doing the exercise on a Swiss ball or wide bench to limit movement at the bottom of the lift (**Fig. 7–14**) will minimize the amount of shoulder extension and horizontal abduction.

This is critically important for patients with anterior GH instability as well as patients who are recovering from anterior stabilization procedures such as open and arthroscopic Bankart and capsulolabral procedures.

Use of a wider grip on the bench press (>2 × biacromial width) results in abduction angles >75 degrees and increases shoulder torques by as much as 1.5 × compared with values with a

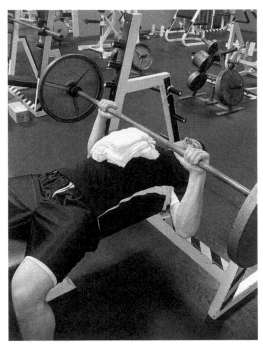

**Figure 7–12** Use of a towel roll on the chest to block the descent phase of the bench press exercise. This serves to limit shoulder extension and horizontal abduction and to minimize anterior capsular stress.

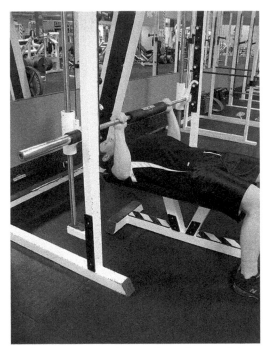

**Figure 7–13** Use of a Smith machine with spot blocks to limit both vertical and horizontal displacement of the bar during a bench press exercise.

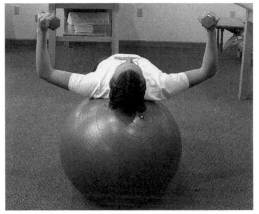

**Figure 7–14** Performance of the bench press on a burst resistant or slow deflate system (SDS) physioball (Hygenic Corporation, Akron, OH) to limit shoulder range of motion and provide proprioceptive cueing during the descent phase of the bench press.

narrower grip.[2] Additionally, the wider grip places great stress on the distal clavicle and should be avoided in patients with AC joint pathology or distal clavicular osteolysis.[2]

In addition to modification of grip and hand position, the bench press can be altered by either raising or lowering the bench, resulting in incline angles of 30 and 45 degrees and decline angles of 15 and 30 degrees. Use of the incline bench press with wider hand positions places the shoulder in a position of abduction and in an ER high-five position; this should be avoided in patients with anterior instability or following anterior stabilization procedures.

Finally, at the top of the movement of the bench press, if scapular dysfunction is present because of serratus anterior weakness, shoulder protraction should be incorporated using a *plus position*, which is characterized by maximal bilateral scapular protraction (**Fig. 7–15**).[16]

### The Cable Fly, the Pec Deck, the Dumbbell Fly, and the Pushup

Other frequently performed chest exercises that place the shoulder in unsafe zones because of the excessive ROM used are the cable fly, the pec deck, the dumbbell fly, and pushup. We will now discuss modifications to these exercises to minimize stress to the shoulder joint and its supporting structures (**Table 7–2**).

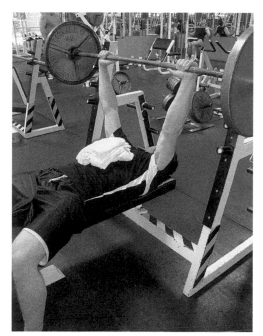

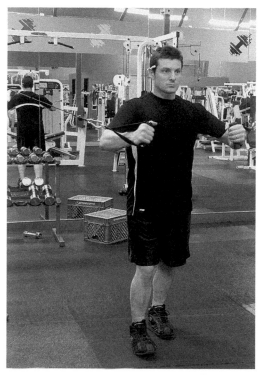

**Figure 7–15** Maximal scapular protraction (the plus position) performed at the end of the bench press exercise to recruit the serratus anterior muscle.

**Figure 7–16** Adjustment of the resistance arm for cable fly exercise, ensuring abduction < 90 degrees while keeping GH joint anterior to the coronal plane at all times.

These traditional chest exercises place excessive stress to the anterior capsulolabral structures of the shoulder, especially when performed posterior to the coronal plane. ROM modifications should be implemented for patients with anterior instability and shoulder impingement when performing these exercises. Special attention to technique must be considered when performing flies on the cable column because of a greater likelihood of variability with technique due to the lack of physical constraints. To decrease anterior shear in performing a cable fly, GH extension and horizontal abduction should not exceed the coronal plane of the body, and actually should remain anterior to the coronal plane during the execution of these exercises. Additionally, GH abduction should be controlled by maintaining the elbow below the level of the shoulder (<90 degrees) and avoiding concomitant internal rotation (IR), which could lead to subacromial impingement. If an adjustable resistance arm is available, the resistance level should be set at or below shoulder level **(Fig. 7–16)**.

The pec deck machine that places the GH joint in the high-five position for at-risk anterior instability patients should be modified by adjusting the start position pads 30 to 45 degrees anterior to the coronal plane. Seat adjustment should be set high to ensure that GH abduction angles remain at <90 degrees during the entire exercise movement pattern **(Fig. 7–17)**.

Dumbbell flies also place excessive stress to the anterior structures of the shoulder, and similar modifications apply with maintaining GH horizontal abduction and extension angles anterior to the coronal plane, while maintaining abduction angles between 45 to 70 degrees to avoid subacromial impingement **(Fig. 7–18)**. To lessen torque about the shoulder, elbow flexion should be maintained between 70 to 90 degrees throughout the movement. An additional modification includes using a physioball instead of a flat bench to limit the amount of shear created posterior to the coronal plane.

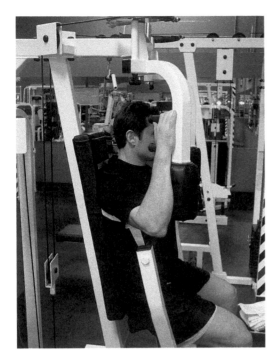

**Figure 7–17** Modification of glenohumeral abduction position on the peck deck to below 90 degrees to minimize the effects of impingement.

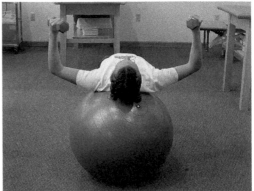

**Figure 7–18** Limitation of shoulder extension and horizontal abduction during the descent phase of the dumbbell fly exercise to protect the anterior capsule of the glenohumeral joint.

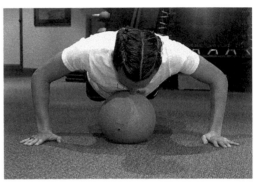

**Figure 7–19** Use of a medicine ball as a barrier to limit the descent phase of the push-up and to minimize the shoulder horizontal abduction stress that is normally present during the traditional, full-ROM push-up.

Similar to the above-mentioned chest exercises with movement beyond the natural resting position of the shoulder, modification of the pushup is necessary for protecting the at-risk shoulder. Limiting hand spacing to <1.5 × the biacromial width lessens anterior shear across the capsule and labrum as well as the AC joint. Glenohumeral abduction angles should be between 45 to 70 degrees while limiting horizontal abduction and extension anterior to the coronal plane. This can be achieved by the use of a medicine ball at sternal level to act as a barrier to motion **(Fig. 7–19)**. In addition, for those individuals with serratus anterior weakness, the plus position of the pushup is a recommended modification.[16] An acceptable modification to the pushup exercise is the step-up. This exercise minimizes the descent phase inherent in the performance of the traditional pushup exercise; yet allows for unilateral shoulder horizontal adduction, elbow extension, and finally toward end ROM maximal scapular protraction to achieve the plus position described by Moseley et al.[16] The step-up exercise is particularly recommended for overhead athletes and for patients following anterior stabilization and rotator cuff disorders.

**The Shoulder Press**

The shoulder press behind the head is not recommended[2,17] because of the anterior shear with the high-five position of the shoulder, as well as increased strain to the cervical region. Additionally, there is an increased risk for subacromial impingement with the shoulders in the full overhead position where dynamic stability is challenged, and the presence of acromial pathology may lead to impingement.[2] The use of dumbbells is recommended over the

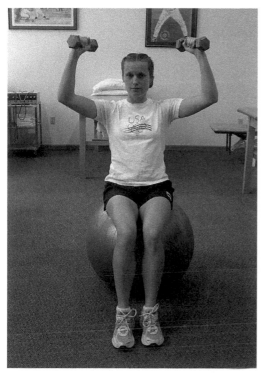

**Figure 7–20** Modification to the shoulder press exercise. Range of motion in the elevation is limited to protect the rotator cuff.

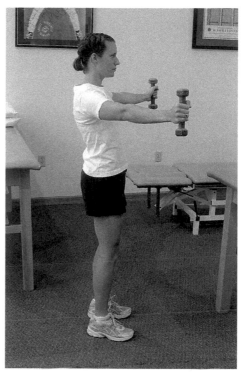

**Figure 7–21** Modification of the lateral raise exercise—scaption (scapular plane elevation) 0–90 degrees.

barbell because of the ability to alter handgrip and shoulder position without having to extend the cervical or lumbar spine for bar clearance. Proper or recommended technique for the modified shoulder press includes a starting position orienting the shoulder(s) in the plane of the scapula, with the forearms in neutral rotation above shoulder level. The exercise motion consists of pushing to three quarters of full range to minimize the effects of GH impingement via subacromial contact (**Fig. 7–20**).

### Lateral Raises and Upright Rows

Lateral raises performed in the coronal plane beyond 90 degrees increase the potential for subacromial impingement because of the lack of obligatory ER that must occur above 90 degrees to clear the greater tuberosity below the acromial arch.[18] Modifications include bringing the resistance into the scapular plane while limiting the movement to <90 degrees into the safe zone (**Fig. 7–21**) (**Table 7–3**).[9]

Upright rows are another exercise to avoid because of the inherent strain to the shoulder with the shoulder maintained in the impingement position (abduction with IR) for over half of the range of movement. The combined movement of shoulder abduction with IR clearly produces impingement and stresses the rotator cuff against the coracoacromial arch. A suggested modification for the targeted muscle—the upper trapezius—would use traditional shoulder shrugs utilizing dumbbells (**Fig. 7–22**).

### Bent-over Rows

To develop the scapular stabilizers and attempt to provide muscular balance to the traditional weightlifting program, which has been historically characterized by exercises targeting anterior muscle groups, the bent-over row is a recommended exercise for patients following shoulder injury or surgery. To limit anterior capsulolabral stress with the bent-over row exercise using a dumbbell, the

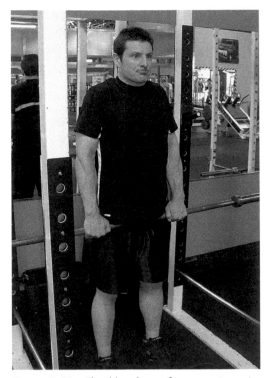

**Figure 7–22** Shoulder shrugs for upper trapezius development.

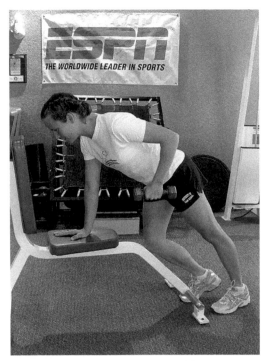

**Figure 7–23** Bent-over row exercise showing proper end-point position with <15 degrees of shoulder extension at end range.

resistance should be maintained close to the body with <30 degrees of GH abduction. Importantly, limiting the end range of the movement to <15 degrees of GH extension is recommended to minimize stress to the anterior capsulolabral structures (**Fig. 7–23**) (**Table 7–4**).

## Overhead Triceps Extension and Dips

Overhead triceps extension is an exercise that should be avoided because of the inherent risk of loading the shoulder in the high-five position behind the coronal plane. Additionally, the elevated humeral position places the GH joint in a position characterized by excessive subacromial contact and stress.[3] A safe alternative to the exercise is the bent-over triceps extension or kickbacks. The starting position maintains the arm in 0 degrees of GH abduction with the elbow flexed to 90 degrees. The exercise movement consists of extending the elbow to full extension without altering the position of the shoulder.

Dips performed through full range of shoulder extension with anterior inclination of the trunk are not recommended for anterior instability or rotator cuff patients because of the stresses imparted to the shoulder, and should be expressly avoided. To best develop the triceps, the exercises in the previous section should be emphasized to target this important muscle while minimizing stress to the GH joint (**Table 7–5**).

## Lattisimus Dorsi Pull-Downs

One of the traditional lifting exercises that exceeds the ROM and stability requirements of the GH joint is the lat pull-down. Traditional performance of this exercise places the shoulder behind the coronal plane of the body with excessive ER of the humerus in addition to promoting an excessive forward head posture stressing the cervical spine (**Fig. 7–24**). This behind the neck pull-down method is a common sight in most gyms and is an unnecessary exercise that should be avoided in individuals

**Table 7–3**  Modifications for Shoulder Exercises: Press, Lateral Raises, and Upright Rows

| Exercise | Pathology | Modifications |
|---|---|---|
| Behind-neck military press (with barbell) | Anterior instability, subacromial impingement, cervical sprain and impingement | • Hand spacing: <1.5 × biacromial width<br>• Resistance brought from posterior→ anterior (in front of head)<br>• ROM limitations: shoulder(s) anterior to coronal plane in scapular plane<br>• End-range position: limiting end-range flexion to ¾ range |
| Shoulder press (dumbbells preferred to barbell with improved control of shoulder position, decreased stress to cervical spine) | Anterior instability, subacromial impingement | • Grip position: neutral rotation<br>• GH position in scapular plane<br>• Start position: slightly above shoulder level<br>• End-range position: limiting end range flexion to ¾ range |
| Lateral raises (with dumbbells) | Subacromial impingement, anterior instability | • Grip position: neutral forearm rotation<br>• GH position in scapular plane<br>• End-range position: <90 degrees |
| Upright rows (with barbell, one or two dumbbells) | Subacromial impingement, AC joint pathology | • Replaced by shoulder shrugs (barbell)<br>• Grip position: overhand grip barbell, neutral rotation with dumbbell(s)<br>• Hand spacing: <1.5 × biacromial width<br>• Movement pattern: Shoulder elevation combined with scapular retraction |

AC, acromioclavicular; GH, glenohumeral, ROM, range of motion.

**Table 7–4**  Modifications for Back Exercises: Latissimus Pull-downs and Bent-over Rows

| Exercise | Pathology | Modifications |
|---|---|---|
| Behind-neck latissimus dorsi pull-downs | Subacromial impingement, anterior instability, long head of biceps pathology, cervical sprain and impingement | • Hand spacing: <1.5 × biacromial width<br>• Movement brought posterior → anterior in front of head, torso reclined 30 degrees<br>• Grip: underhand, overhand, and neutral (variation based on pathology)<br>• GH abduction angles maintained in scapular plane<br>• Limit overhead arm position ¾ range decreasing subacromial impingement<br>• Emphasize scapular retraction from mid → late concentric phase of lift |
| Bent-over rows (dumbbell) | Anterior instability, subacromial impingement | • Grip: neutral<br>• ROM limitations: GH abduction <30 degrees, shoulder extension anterior to coronal plane at top of movement |

GH, glenohumeral, ROM, range of motion.

**Table 7–5**  Modifications for Overhead Triceps Extensions and Dips

| Exercise | Pathology | Modifications |
|---|---|---|
| Behind-head triceps extension (dumbbell) | Anterior instability, subacromial impingement | • Substitution exercise: triceps kickback<br>• Start position: similar to bent-over row<br>• ROM limitations: GH abduction <30 degrees, extension anterior to coronal plane |
| Front dips on dip bar | Anterior instability, subacromial impingement | • Substitution exercise: Alternate triceps exercise<br>• Note: Exercise not recommended for patients recovering from shoulder injury because of difficulty in maintaining necessary ROM limitations |

GH, glenohumeral, ROM, range of motion.

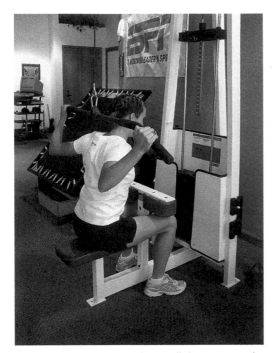

**Figure 7–24** Latissimus dorsi pull-downs. Note the forward head position and high-five position of abduction and external rotation of the shoulders inherent in this "behind-the-head" technique.

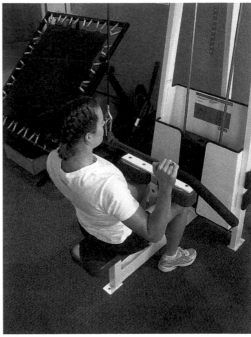

**Figure 7–25** Latissimus dorsi pull-downs showing "in-front-of-head" technique. Also recommended is the shoulder-width grip, shoulders positioned in scapular plane, scapula retracted, limiting three-quarters flexion range, and elbows flexed ~30 degrees.

with a history of shoulder pathology.[2] Reports of transient upper-extremity paralysis have been reported following execution of this exercise. In addition, it places stresses on the rotator cuff and capsular restraint mechanisms of the GH joint.[19]

The primary modification of this exercise involves movement of the bar toward the chest in front of the head, which is done by reclining the torso ~30 degrees (**Fig. 7–25**) (**Table 7–4**). Recommended grip widths are 1.25 to 1.5 × the biacromial width. In addition to being safer, the front lat pull-down exercise has been shown to have an inherent advantage of greater scapular retraction and shoulder adduction than the traditional behind the neck variation of this exercise.[2] Electromyogram (EMG) research has shown that greater muscular activity of the scapular retractors and shoulder adductors exists with the front pull-down variation with a contact point of the bar just proximal to the xiphoid process of the sternum.

Finally, during the lat pull exercise, care must be taken during the eccentric return of the bar to the overhead position. Rapid, uncontrolled movements may result in a flexion overpressure movement that is an additional item of caution with this exercise. Limiting the range of overhead return not only can protect the rotator cuff from impingement, but also can increase the eccentric function of the shoulder adductor musculature, thus adding to the effectiveness of this exercise for that muscle group.

### ◆ Ramifications of Lower Extremity Exercise on the Shoulder

Although it is beyond the scope of this chapter to outline all of the potentially harmful positions and ramifications of traditional lower extremity exercises on the upper extremity, it

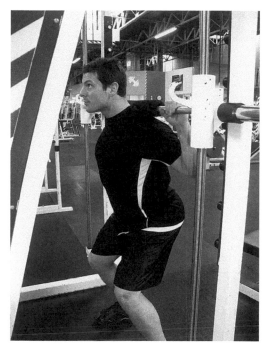

**Figure 7–26** Traditional squat position loading the anterior shoulder structures.

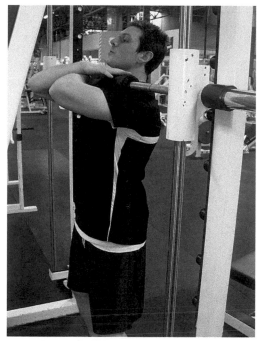

**Figure 7–27** Alternative to the traditional squat position, the front squat places the shoulder in a more neutral position to allow the loading on the lower extremity during exercise.

is important to realize that the concepts developed regarding the safe zone should apply to all lifting activities in the gym, not just those that focus on the chest and upper body.[20] One particularly common exercise that can create significant shoulder loads is the behind-the-back squat.

### Behind-the-Back Squats

Behind the back squats, especially a "low bar" resting position,[2] places increased stress to the shoulder because of the high-five position of the shoulder necessary to stabilize the weight (**Fig. 7–26**). An alternative to the back squat is the front squat, where the bar is placed anteriorly on the anterior deltoids and sternoclavicular joints with the shoulder in 80 to 90 degrees of flexion and <15 degrees of ER resulting in decreased stress to the middle and inferior GH ligaments (**Fig. 7–27**). Patients returning to their exercise program following surgery should perform this lower-extremity exercise strategy to stabilize the capsulolabral structures and rotator cuff repair. Overhead

athletes to avoid undue stress to the capsulolabral structures should also follow this lower-extremity exercise strategy.

### ◆ Summary

Many of the traditional upper-extremity lifts (bench press, military press, pull-downs) performed by the recreational weightlifter, bodybuilder, and athlete create potentially harmful forces to the shoulder complex when the ROM exceeds the static and dynamic stability of the shoulder. When individuals recovering from shoulder injury or surgery perform these exercises, it is necessary to modify these lifts to prevent reinjury to the shoulder from undue stress. We have discussed several of the more common exercises along with specific modifications to lessen the potentially harmful forces. It is advised that when returning to these exercises with the necessary modifications to consult with your rehabilitation professional.

# References

1. Gross ML, Brenner SL, Esformes I, Sonogni JJ. Anterior shoulder instability in weight lifters. Am J Sports Med 1993;21:599–603

2. Fees M, Decker T, Snyder-Mackler L, Axe MJ. Upper extremity weight training modifications for the injured athlete. Am J Sports Med 1998;26:732–742

3. Wuelker N, Plitz W, Roetman B. Biomechanical data concerning the shoulder impingement syndrome. Clin Orthop Relat Res 1994;303:242–249

4. Lucas DB. Biomechanics of the shoulder joint. Arch Surg 1973;107:425–432

5. Zuckerman JD, Kummer FJ, Cuomo F, et al. The influence of coracoacromial arch anatomy on rotator cuff tears. J Shoulder Elbow Surg 1992;1:4–14

6. Bigliani LU, Ticker JB, Flatow EL, Soslowsky LJ, Mow VC. The relationship of acromial architecture to rotator cuff disease. Clin Sports Med 1991;10:823–838

7. O'Brien SJ, Beves MC, Arnoczky SJ, et al. The anatomy and histology of the inferior glenohumeral ligament complex of the shoulder. Am J Sports Med 1990;18:449–456

8. Wilk KE, Arrigo AA, Andrews JR. Current concepts: the stabilizing structures of the glenohumeral joint. J Orthop Sports Phys Ther 1997;25:364–379

9. Ellenbecker, TS. Postrehabilitation shoulder conditioning for tennis. IDEA Personal Trainer 2000;11:18–27

10. Norkin CC, Levangie PK. Joint Structure and Function: A Comprehensive Analysis. 2nd ed. Philadelphia: FA Davis; 1992

11. Saha AK. Mechanism of shoulder movements and a plea for the recognition of "zero position" of glenohumeral joint. Clin Orthop Relat Res 1983;173:3–10

12. Baechle TR. Essentials of Strength Training and Conditioning. Champaign, IL: Human Kinetics; 1994

13. Banas MP, Miller RJ, Totterman S. Relationship between the lateral acromion angle and rotator cuff disease. J Shoulder Elbow Surg 1995;4:454–461

14. Corso G. Impingement relief test: an adjunctive procedure to traditional assessment of shoulder impingement syndrome. J Orthop Sports Phys Ther 1995;22:183–192

15. Barnett C, Kippers V, Turner P. Effects of variations of the bench press exercise on the EMG activity of fiver shoulder muscles. J Strength Cond Res 1995;(9)4:222–227

16. Moseley JB Jr, Jobe FW, Pink M, et al. EMG analysis of the scapular muscles during a shoulder rehabilitation program. Am J Sports Med 1992;20:128–134

17. Brumitt, JB. Exercise modifications for shoulder instability. National Strength and Conditioning. Association Performance Training Journal 2005; 4:9–10

18. Poppen NK, Walker PS. Forces at the glenohumeral joint in abduction. Clin Orthop Relat Res 1978;135:165–170

19. Shea JM. Acute quadriplegia following use of progressive resistance exercise machinery: a case report. Phys Sportsmed 1986;12:120–124

20. Durall CJ, Manske RC, Davies GJ. Avoiding shoulder injury from resistance training. J Strength and Conditioning 2001;23:10–18

# 8

# Use of Taping and External Devices in Shoulder Rehabilitation

**Anna E. Thatcher and George J. Davies**

The glenohumeral (GH) joint is an inherently unstable joint and injuries are often related to or result in a decrease in joint stability. Many of the shoulder pathologies discussed in this book are influenced by improper GH and scapulothoracic (ST) biomechanics. In addition to the strengthening and proprioceptive exercises discussed in previous chapters, external devices such as taping and bracing are used clinically in an attempt to increase shoulder stability and improve function. The lack of stable structures in the shoulder joint makes it more difficult to stabilize with tape or a brace than the knee and ankle joints. Compared with the studies on taping and bracing lower extremity joints,[1-5] there is considerably less research on taping and bracing the shoulder complex. In this chapter, we will summarize the current literature on the use of shoulder taping and bracing in the nonoperative treatment of shoulder pathologies.

## ◆ Shoulder Taping

### Clinical Rationale for the Use of Shoulder Taping

The purpose of taping is to provide protection and support for a joint while still allowing necessary movement for sport activities.[6] Tape is believed to have both mechanical and proprioceptive effects that assist in improving shoulder stability, correcting faulty biomechanics and posture, and ultimately decreasing pain and increasing function. There are numerous clinical assumptions on why tape may be effective in decreasing subjective complaints of pain and increasing function (**Table 8–1**).

According to Morrisey,[7] taping methods may be used to inhibit or activate muscles. When tape is applied under tension in the direction of lengthened muscle fibers, it is thought to facilitate underlying muscle contraction by shortening the muscle. As the lengthened muscle becomes shortened, the length–tension relationship is optimized and maximal muscle contraction is possible.[16] Tape applied to lengthen a shortened muscle is thought to inhibit the muscle. It is theorized tape may increase afferent input that will decrease volitional drive to the motor neuron pool from the descending pathways, resulting in muscle inhibition.[8] Although taping may

**Table 8–1**  Clinical Assumptions on Why Shoulder Taping Is Effective

- Varies the muscle length–tension relationship to facilitate or inhibit muscle activation[7]
- Provides cutaneous receptor stimulation[6-9]
- Alters subjective sense of muscle contraction[8]
- Provides proprioceptive feedback[7,10]
- Promotes proximal scapular stability through biomechanical realignment[10-12]
- Restores normal glenohumeral function[13]
- Changes muscle reaction times[6]
- Improves posture/postural awareness[6,14]
- Increases subjective parameters of comfort[6]
- Allows a low load, prolonged stretch to soft tissue structures[10]
- Unloads painful structures[11]
- Psychological effects[15]

decrease subjective complaints of pain and improve function as a result of any combination of the above factors, much of the rationale for shoulder taping is based on anecdotal clinical reports.[10-12,17-19] As discussed later in this chapter, there is no strong evidence to support shoulder taping in the current scientific literature.

### Methods of Shoulder Taping

Clinicians use tape as an adjunct to other non-operative methods of treating various shoulder pathologies.[10-12,17-19] Methods of shoulder taping have been described in the treatment of shoulder impingement,[10,20] multidirectional instability[11] and laxity,[9] acromioclavicular (AC) joint sprains,[19,20] GH subluxation due to underlying neurologic injury,[21,22] and to improve posture.[20,21] We will describe the use of tape in the treatment of multidirectional instability, anterior instability, scapular stabilization, and AC joint sprains.

#### General Taping Instructions

- Skin in the area to be taped is cleaned to remove any lotions, oils, etc. If desired, adhesive taping spray may be used.
- The patient sits in an upright posture with the scapula and GH joint actively or passively held in the desired position.

- An undertape (i.e., Hypafix; Smith & Nephew Healthcare Ltd., Hull, UK) is used to minimize skin irritation.
- A rigid tape (i.e., Leukotape; 3M, Maplewood, MN) is placed over the undertape. This tape is applied under tension in the desired direction to support the shoulder.

### Multidirectional Shoulder Instability Taping Instructions

Three strips of tape are applied in an attempt to stabilize the GH joint. This taping procedure was used in the study by Hiltbrand et al[9] and is pictured in **Figure 8–1**.

1. Place a pillow under the arm to position the GH joint in slight abduction.
2. Begin with tape over the anterior aspect of proximal humerus and pull superiorly, anchoring tape over the posterior shoulder.
3. Place a second strip of tape over the middle aspect of the proximal humerus and anchor over the superior shoulder.
4. The third strip of tape begins over the posterior aspect of the proximal humerus and ends over the anterosuperior shoulder.

### Anterior Instability Taping Instructions

This taping procedure is used in patients with pathologies related to anterior instability. One or more strips of tape are applied in an attempt to stabilize the humeral head (**Fig. 8–2**).

1. Begin by anchoring tape over anterior aspect of the humeral head. Passively apply a slight posterior force to the humeral head, pull tape over top of shoulder, and anchor medial to the inferior scapular border.
2. Repeat as needed, beginning each strip of tape overlapping the previous one.

### Scapular Stabilization Taping Instructions

Several variations of taping to stabilize the scapula and normalize scapulohumeral rhythm are described in the literature.[6,7,10,12,15,20,24,25] Similar taping variations are also described as an attempt to inhibit the upper trapezius muscle and/or maximize activation of the lower trapezius muscle.[7,8,15,26] The taping method for scapular stabilization described by Cools et al[6] and Morrisey[7] is presented in **Figure 8–3**.

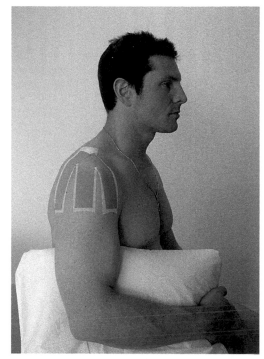

**Figure 8–1**  Taping procedure for multidirectional instability.

1. Begin tape over anterior shoulder, just below the coracoid process.
2. Pull superiorly and then posteriorly on the tape to anchor over the lower thoracic area.

### Acromioclavicular Joint Taping Instructions

Various taping methods to stabilize the AC joint after an injury have been described in the literature.[15,19,20,27] The method pictured in **Figure 8–4** was found to be effective at decreasing pain and contributed to range of motion (ROM) and strength improvements in a published case report.[19]

1. The patient's elbow should be supported and an approximation force applied to the shoulder joint to move the humerus superiorly.
2. Begin the first strip of tape over the middle deltoid and pull upward to anchor tape proximal to the AC joint. Tape should not interfere with the upper trapezius muscle belly.
3. The second strip of tape is applied from the coracoid process to the spine of the scapula.

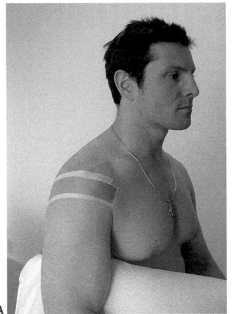
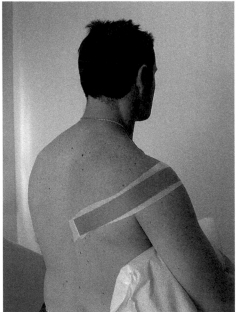

**A**

**B**

**Figure 8–2** **(A)** Anterior view of taping procedure for anterior instability. **(B)** Posterior view of taping procedure for anterior instability.

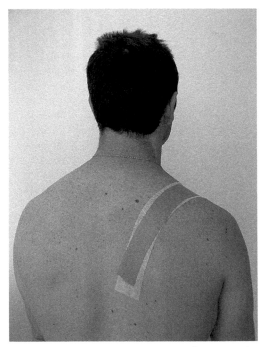

**Figure 8–3** Taping procedure for scapular stabilization.

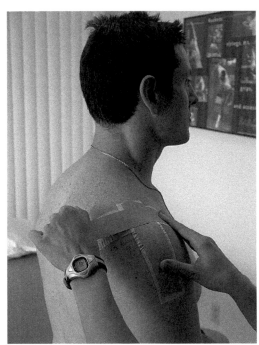

**Figure 8–4** Taping procedure for the acromioclavicular joint.

## Effectiveness of Shoulder Taping in Orthopaedic Conditions

Although shoulder taping is frequently used as an adjunct to treat and prevent shoulder injuries, its effectiveness has not been well studied in the published literature. Case studies that have been found present anecdotal evidence for the use of shoulder taping in the treatment of a variety of shoulder pathologies, including impingement,[10-12] AC joint sprains,[19] shoulder subluxation secondary to neurologic disorders,[18] and chronic shoulder dislocations exacerbating symptoms of reflex sympathetic dystrophy.[17] In all of these case studies, tape was used as an adjunct to other methods of conservative treatment, including modalities, postural education, and rotator cuff and scapular muscle strengthening. The authors noted symptom relief and improved shoulder function and attributed these outcomes to the tape application. However, the use of multiple interventions in most studies makes it difficult to attribute the results to shoulder taping alone.

Despite the positive outcomes with taping presented in these case studies, there is no consensus on the effect of shoulder taping in research studies. It is difficult to summarize and compare the current literature because of the use of various taping methods and outcome measures. Research on the effects of shoulder taping on scapular muscle activity, GH joint proprioception, impingement, and joint laxity secondary to neurologic disorders is discussed below. The results are summarized in **Table 8–2**.

### Orthopaedic Applications

Three published research studies have investigated the effects of shoulder taping on ST muscle activity in healthy shoulders. The two most comparable research studies were done by Morin et al[26] and Cools et al[6] to determine the effectiveness of tape on inhibiting the upper trapezius muscles. In both studies, tape was applied by starting on the anterior shoulder, pulling firmly over the upper trapezius, and attaching the tape medial to the scapula at a lower thoracic level. Morin et al[26] found taping did inhibit the upper trapezius muscle and increased middle/lower trapezius muscle activity during isometric contractions. In contrast to these beneficial effects, Cools et al[6] found taping had no significant effect on the electromyographic (EMG) activity of the trapezius (upper, middle, and lower) or serratus anterior muscles during dynamic movements. Although EMG results are less steady during dynamic movements than isometric contractions, dynamic movements are more functional and clinically relevant.[6]

Ackermann et al[24] investigated the effect of tape on muscle activity in string musicians during functional activity. Tape applied as described by Morrisey[7] to increase scapular retraction and upward rotation was found to have no effect on scapular rotator muscle activity and actually increased upper trapezius activity. In addition, taping had the negative effects of decreasing comfort, concentration, and performance quality as reported by the violinists. The authors suggest more positive results may occur if tape was repeatedly applied so subjects could become accustomed to the tape. Also, repeated tape application may allow for adaptation of neural pathways.

Some of the strongest anecdotal evidence for shoulder taping is based on its presumed ability to stimulate cutaneous receptors and improve proprioceptive and kinesthetic awareness. Research on this hypothesis includes two studies investigating the effect of shoulder taping on joint reposition sense. Zanella et al[25] found scapular taping had no effect on shoulder joint reposition sense. This was true for shoulders with and without scapular winging. Hiltbrand et al[9] investigated the effects of McConnell taping on joint-reposition sense in shoulders with and without multidirectional GH joint laxity. Results showed an increase in accuracy of joint position sense by 1.449 degrees in flexion and 1.221 degrees in abduction when the tape was applied. Although this increase in joint-position sense was statistically significant, the clinical significance of a goniometric measurement of <2 degrees was questioned by the authors.

Research by Lewis et al[14] and Page and Stewart[13] investigated the effect of shoulder taping in subjects with primary and secondary impingement, respectively. Lewis et al[14] examined the effects of changing posture on shoulder ROM in subjects with and without primary subacromial impingement. Changes in shoulder pain were also evaluated in the

**Table 8–2**  Summary of Published Research Studies on the Effectiveness of Shoulder Taping

| Author | Subject Description | Number of Subjects | Clinical Goal of Taping Method Used | Method of Assessment | Did Taping Achieve the Clinical Goal? |
|---|---|---|---|---|---|
| Ackermann et al[24] | Professional violinists performing musical excerpts | 8 | Improvement in scapular position and shoulder muscle efficiency | Surface EMG of upper trapezius and scapular retractors | No; upper trapezius muscle activation was increased. |
| Alexander et al[8] | Healthy subjects | 18 | Facilitation of lower trapezius muscle | Surface EMG of lower trapezius | No; lower trapezius muscle activation was inhibited. |
| Cools et al[6] | Healthy subjects performing AROM abduction and flexion | 20 | Alter activation of trapezius and serratus anterior muscles | Surface EMG of trapezius and serratus anterior muscles | No; activation of upper, middle, lower trapezius or serratus anterior muscles was not significantly changed. |
| Hanger et al[21] | Subjects with an acute hemiplegic stroke and shoulder abduction weakness | 98 | Decrease pain, maintain ROM, and improve functional outcomes after cerebrovascular accidents | Visual Analog Scale for pain, shoulder ROM, Functional Independence Measure, Motor Assessment Scale, Rankin Disability Index, | No; there was a trend toward achieving the clinical goals but it did not reach statistical significance. |
| Lewis et al[14] | Subjects with primary impingement | 120 | Static postural changes | Forward head and shoulder posture, shoulder ROM, Visual Analog Scale for pain | Yes; static posture was improved; some subjects had improved ROM. |
| Morin et al[26] | Healthy subjects performing isometric contractions | 10 | Alter activation of upper and middle/lower trapezius | Surface EMG of trapezius muscle | Yes; upper trapezius activation decreased and middle/lower trapezius activation increased. |
| Morin and Bravo[22] | Hemiplegic subjects | 15 | Decrease shoulder subluxation after cerebrovascular accident | Radiographic evaluation of subluxation | Yes; use of sling and taping decreased shoulder subluxation. |
| Zanella et al[25] | Asymptomatic subjects with and without scapular winging | 36 | Improve active shoulder joint reposition sense | Error in joint repositioning with active flexion and abduction on isokinetic dynamometer | No; taping had no effect on reposition sense. |

AROM, active range of motion; EMG, electromyography; ROM, range of motion.

symptomatic subjects. Tape was applied over the thoracic spine in an attempt to create a postural change. With the scapula in a position of retraction and depression and the thoracic spine extended, tape was placed from T1 to T12 and from the spine of the scapula to T12. Results showed taping did produce favorable static postural changes including decreased forward head posture, forward shoulder posture, and thoracic kyphosis in both symptomatic and asymptomatic subjects. This study does not give any evidence that posture during movement was altered by the taping technique. Taping allowed greater ROM before the onset of pain in symptomatic subjects; however, the intensity of pain when it did occur was not reduced. The authors suggested future studies investigate the long-term effects of taping and the characteristics of subjects who will benefit from taping because not every subject responded favorably.

Page and Stewart[13] investigated the effects of taping on secondary impingement. Subjects included were recreational athletes with laxity of the GH joint capsule and positive impingement testing. The authors found that shoulder taping, in addition to rotator cuff strengthening, scapular stabilization exercises, and posture education was effective in decreasing pain and improving function in subjects with secondary impingement. Subjects were seen for 7 to 20 visits and returned to athletic activity after 2 to 8 weeks of treatment. No other specific data was included in this abstract.

Mulligan[23] (unpublished data) has also researched the use of tape to optimize shoulder position and possibly improve shoulder function. Subjects in this study were high school baseball pitchers with and without scapular muscle weakness. Isokinetic strength and pitch velocity were tested in all subjects with and without a taping technique to place the humerus in a posterior position. Results showed improvement in external rotation (ER) to internal rotation (IR) strength ratios and pitch velocity in subjects with and without scapular weakness when the taping procedure was applied. Subjects with scapular weakness had an increase in pitch velocity from 65.72 miles per hour to 67.24 miles per hour after tape was applied. Pitch velocity increased from 69.88 to 71.44 after tape was applied in subjects without scapular weakness. There were

no significant improvements in strength or pitch velocity in either group with a placebo taping procedure; hence, the author hypothesizes the improvements seen are because the tape had a stabilizing effect on the ST articulation and optimized the biomechanics of the shoulder complex.

### Neurologic Applications

In addition to its use in treating orthopedic conditions, shoulder taping has been shown to be effective in reducing subluxation secondary to neurologic disorders. The combination of shoulder taping and use of a sling had a greater effect on reducing subluxation in hemiplegic shoulders than either intervention separately.[22] Although not statistically significant, Hanger et al[21] found a trend toward decreased pain, preservation of ROM, and improved functional outcomes in hemiplegic patients with shoulder abduction weakness that underwent shoulder taping.

## ◆ Shoulder Braces

### Use of Shoulder Braces in Return to Athletic Activity

Although not as commonly prescribed as knee and ankle braces, shoulder braces are used during sports participation. Braces are used prophylactically in returning athletes to sport with the goal of increasing GH joint stability. By limiting abduction and ER, a brace could potentially prevent anterior glenohumeral dislocations, which account for the majority of recurrent dislocations. Factors related to a brace's ability to limit ROM include the restraint system (i.e., laces, plastic clips), deformation of composition materials, and brace–body interface.[28] Similar to shoulder taping, braces have not only mechanical but also proprioceptive effects to minimize joint injury.

### Examples of Shoulder Braces Used during Athletic Activity

Braces vary in design characteristics and capability to limit different motions; therefore, the individual athlete and sport need to be considered to

**Table 8–3**   Classification of Sport Types Based on Shoulder Demands

| Type | Functional Description | Athlete | Forces on Shoulder |
|------|------------------------|---------|--------------------|
| I | Skilled overhead use, full ROM required | Thrower, swimmer, racket sports player, golfer | Overhead use, primarily acceleration and repetitive motion |
| II | Skilled overhead use (nonthrowers), full ROM required | Wide-receiver, basketball rebounder, volleyball blocker, gymnast | Overhead use, primarily deceleration |
| IIIA | High-impact forces, full ROM required | Linebacker, defensive linemen, soccer goalkeeper | Direct blow or strain placed on shoulder |
| IIIB | High-impact forces, full ROM not required | Hockey defense, offensive lineman, soccer striker, water sports | Direct blow or strain placed on shoulder |

Source: From O'Brien SJ, Warren RF, Schwartz E. Anterior shoulder instability. Orthop Clin North Am 1987;18: 395–408. Also reprinted in Reuss BL, Harding WG III, Nowicki KD. Managing anterior shoulder instability with bracing: an expanded update. Orthopedics 2004;27:614–618. Reprinted here by permission.

ROM, range of motion.

determine the most appropriate brace. A thorough review of functional shoulder braces for athletes with anterior shoulder instability was published by Reuss et al.[29] The authors provide a classification system of sports based on shoulder demands (see **Table 8–3**). Thirteen shoulder braces are described, including supplier, comfort, cosmesis, ease of application, and special features (refer to **Tables 8–4** and **8–5**).[29] Examples of three shoulder braces commonly used for athletes with shoulder instability are shown in **Figures 8–5 to 8–7**. In addition to bracing for instability, a scapula winger's brace has been described in the management of long thoracic nerve palsy.[34]

### Evidence-Based Effectiveness of Shoulder Braces

Current research on the effectiveness of shoulder braces has investigated injury recurrence rates, motion restriction, and joint reposition sense. Clinical observations by Sawa[35] report no injury recurrence after GH subluxation or dislocation in hockey players following a three-phase rehabilitation program. The three phases included: (1) rest and nutrition, (2) interferential current and muscle stimulation, and (3) a traditional progressive-resistance weight-training program in conjunction with a shoulder orthosis. The author feels these three phases help optimize the natural healing process after injury. The orthosis

used permitted variable restriction of shoulder abduction, allowing controlled movement within safe ranges of motion. The above clinical observations suggest use of a shoulder orthosis during the healing process to optimize shoulder rehabilitation and decrease injury recurrence rates. Sawa[35] reports further scientific research is needed to determine the specific role of the orthosis in the healing process.

Two published research studies have investigated the effect of braces on limiting shoulder passive and/or active ROM. DeCarlo et al[31] studied the effects of three shoulder braces, Sawa (DonJoy/dj Orthopedics, Inc., Vista, CA), Duke Wyre (CD Denison Orthopaedic Appliance Corp., Baltimore, MD), and Shoulder Subluxation Inhibitor (Boston Brace International, Inc., Avon, MA), on limiting active motion following isokinetic exercise. All three braces did exhibit a loosening effect and allowed a significant increase in flexion ROM after exercise. However, a significant increase in ER was not allowed by any of the braces. The Duke Wyre and Shoulder Subluxation Inhibitor braces were also effective in limiting abduction. Because it allows flexion ROM and limits abduction, the authors suggest the Shoulder Subluxation Inhibitor brace may be useful for sporting activities that require overhead movements.

Weise et al[28] found similar effects when investigating the Duke Wyre and Sawa

**Table 8–4** Description of Shoulder Braces

| Name (Supplier) | Comfort, Cosmesis, Ease of Application | Construction/Adjustment | Special Features | Potential Sport Use (Type) |
|---|---|---|---|---|
| Acro Comfort (Otto Bock, Minneapolis, MN) | Comfortable, cosmetically pleasing, requires no assistance to apply | Polyester; hook and loop fastener for direct humeral head force in anteroposterior or axial direction | Contains "Phase Change Materials" for temperature control; washable | I, II, IIIA, IIIB |
| Cadlow Shoulder Stabilizer (DM Systems, Inc., Evanston, IL) | Comfortable, cosmetically pleasing, requires no assistance to apply, initial assembly is time consuming, requires McDavid compression shorts that hook into brace | Canvas straps with felt padding and adjustment bungee cords attached to arm strap; McDavid compression shorts attach to brace via hooks | Uses series of adjustable bungee cords to maintain shoulder in safe zone (dynamically); allows increased ROM by using lower tension bungee cords, shorts prevent brace migration; washable | I, II, IIIA, IIIB |
| Curtis Shoulder Cuff (EBI Medical Systems, Inc., Parsippany, NJ) | Comfortable, requires no assistance to apply | Neoprene/hook and loop fastener with adjustable canvas straps | Washable | IIIB |
| Duke Wyre Shoulder Vest (CD Denison Orthopaedic Appliance Corp., Baltimore, MD) | Satisfactory, requires minimal assistance first application | Canvas, leather with adjustable shoestrings to statically control abduction and extension but not ER | Dry clean only | IIIB |
| OmoTrain (Bauerfeind, Kennesaw, GA) | Comfortable, cosmetically pleasing, requires no assistance to apply | Bi-elastic knitted support, elastic straps through plastic loops for adjustment | Allows full ROM with minimal ability to restrict motion/stabilize, washable | I, II, IIIA, IIIB |
| Shoulder Controller (Professional's Choice Sports Medicine Products, Inc., El Cajon, CA) | Comfortable, cosmetically pleasing, requires no assitance to apply | Neoprene/spandex with elastic and hook and loop fastener to adjust direct, dynamic anterior or posterior humeral head force | Allows full ROM, compression straps allow for pads/ice packs to be placed, washable | I, II, IIIA, IIIB |
| Shoulder Stability Brace (Medco Supply Co., Tonawanda, NY) | Comfortable, cosmetically pleasing, requires minimal assistance to apply | Neoprene with adjustable elastic hook and loop fastener | Can be used on either shoulder, both anterior and posterior direct humeral head compression along with indirect support in abduction and extension; washable | I, II, IIIA, IIIB |
| Shoulder Stabilizer (BREG, Inc., Vista, CA) | Comfortable, cosmetically pleasing, requires minimal assistance to apply | Neoprene/hook and loop fastener with adjustable canvas straps through plastic loops for static abduction and extension control | Washable | IIIB |

| Name (Supplier) | Comfort, Cosmesis, Ease of Application | Construction/ Adjustment | Special Features | Potential Sport Use (Type) |
|---|---|---|---|---|
| Sawa/Shoulder Stabilizer (DonJoy/dj Orthopedics, Inc., Vista, CA) | Comfortable, cosmetically pleasing, requires no assistance to apply | Polyester/lycra with adjustable hook and loop fastener for restriction in extension, external rotation or abduction | Adjustable rigid control, axillary strap provides direct humeral head compression or AC compression for AC joint sprains, can be used on either shoulder, washable | II, IIIA, IIIB |
| Shoulder Subluxation Inhibitor (Boston Brace International, Inc., Avon, MA) | Satisfactory, requires minimal assistance to apply, requires initial assembly with Loctite tool for proper fit | Rigid polyethylene, elastic straps with buckle adjustment, custom fit | Allows full ROM or can be adjusted to limit abduction and extension, rigid polyethylene may be beneficial in contact sports | II, IIIA, IIIB |
| Simply Shoulder Stabilizer (Seattle Systems, Poulsbo, WA) | Comfortable, requires no assistance to apply, sternal plate can be compressive on large chested individuals | Neoprene/hook and loop fastener, adjustable strap | Can be attached directly to shoulder pads instead of sternal plate harness, can be used on either shoulder, washable | II, IIIA, IIIB |
| Sully (The Saunders Group, Inc., Chaska, MN) | Comfortable, cosmetically pleasing, requires no assistance to apply | Neoprene with adjustable elastic hook and loop fastener | ROM can be restricted in abduction; allows full ER and extension, washable | I, II, IIIA, IIIB |
| Universal Shoulder Support (McDavid Sports/ Medical Products, Woodridge, IL) | Comfortable, cosmetically pleasing, requires minimal assistance to apply | Neoprene with accessory hook and loop fastener to restrict either anterior or posterior instability | Pocket over shoulder can be used to insert pad for direct compression, washable | I, II, IIIA, IIIB |

Source: From Reuss BL, Harding WG III, Nowicki KD. Managing anterior shoulder instability with bracing: an expanded update. Orthopedics 2004;27:614–618. Reprinted by permission.

AC, acromioclavicular; ER, external rotation; ROM, range of motion.

**Table 8–5**  Summary of Published Research Studies on the Effectiveness of Shoulder Braces

| Author | Shoulder Brace(s) | Subject Description | Number of Subjects | Clinical Goal of Bracing | Method of Assessment | Did Brace Achieve the Clinical Goal? |
|---|---|---|---|---|---|---|
| Chu et al[30] | Neoprene Shoulder Stabilizer (Sully Shoulder Stabilizer) | Subjects with and without prior history of dislocation | 40 | Improve active joint-reposition sense | IR and ER joint-reposition sense isokinetic on dynamometer | Yes; Even though the brace did not limit ER motion, active joint-reposition sense was improved in unstable shoulders. |
| DeCarlo et al[31] | Sawa, Duke Wyre, Shoulder Subluxation Inhibitor | Healthy subjects | 10 | Limit active ROM after exercise | Active ROM measured by goniometer | Yes; ER was limited by all three braces, abduction was limited by the Duke Wyre and the Shoulder Subluxation Inhibitor. |
| Ulkar et al[32] | Neoprene sleeve | Healthy subjects | 26 | Improve passive joint-reposition sense | Prosport 1000 PMS (device for measuring passive joint-reposition sense and threshold to detection of passive motion) | Yes; bracing improved passive joint-reposition sense. |
| Walther et al[33] | Coopercare-Lastrap Functional Shoulder Brace | Subjects with subacromial impingement | 60 | Relieve symptoms | Visual Analog Scale for pain, Constant-Murley score | Yes; Bracing had similar results to self-training and conventional physical therapy. |
| Weise et al[28] | Denison and Duke Wyre Harness, Sawa Shoulder Brace | Healthy subjects | 15 | Limit active and passive range of motion | Angular displacement measured by PEAK Motus motion analysis system | No; Preset brace limits were not maintained; however, the shoulder was protected from reaching a position of 90 degrees abduction and ER. |

ER, external rotation; IR, internal rotation; ROM, range of motion.

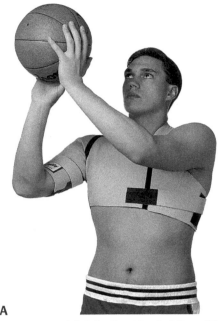

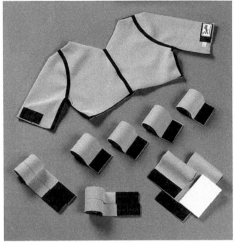

**A**

**B**

**Figure 8–5** **(A)** Sully Shoulder Stabilizer. **(B)** Sully Shoulder Stabilizer–Bilateral. (Illustrations used with the permission of The Saunders Group, Inc., Chaska, MN.)

shoulder braces. Although neither brace maintained its preset limit of 45 degrees abduction during active or passive joint movement, both braces effectively prohibited the shoulder from actively reaching the vulnerable position of 90 degrees abduction and 90 degrees ER where dislocations are likely to occur. These two braces also limited passive abduction to <90 degrees and the Sawa brace limited passive ER to <90 degrees. Passive ROM is important to consider because passive forces can

cause injury during contact sports. Published abstracts agree with the findings of the above studies that shoulder braces loosen with shoulder movement and do not restrict active ROM to preset limits.[36,37]

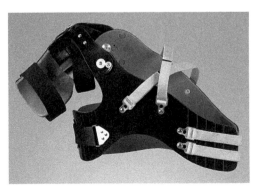

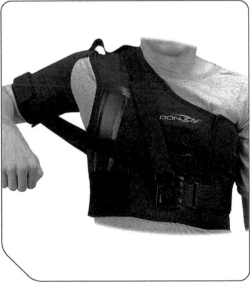

**Figure 8–6** Unilateral Shoulder Subluxation Inhibitor. (Used with permission from Boston Brace International, Inc., Avon, MA.)

**Figure 8–7** Shoulder Stabilizer (DonJoy). (Used with permission from dj Orthopedics, LLC, Vista, CA.)

Although shoulder braces may not significantly limit ROM, there is evidence they improve proprioception. A study by Chu et al[30] found active joint-reposition sense near end-range ER in unstable shoulders to be significantly improved when wearing a neoprene shoulder brace (Sully Shoulder Stabilizer; The Saunders Group Inc, Chaska, MN). Results for unstable shoulders showed joint-reposition sense absolute mean error scores at 10 degrees from full ER improved from 8.37 degrees (±1.3) in the unbraced condition to 4.55 degrees (±0.65) in the braced condition. The authors attributed this finding to increased cutaneous input because the brace had no effect on limiting shoulder ER. When worn by subjects with stable shoulders, the brace had no effect on joint-reposition sense; however, it did limit ER. Neoprene shoulder braces have also been found to improve passive joint-position sense. Ulkar et al[32] used a proprioception measurement device (Prosport 1000 PMS; Tümer Engineering Co. Ltd., Ankara, Turkey) to evaluate the effect of a neoprene shoulder brace on passive position sense at 45 degrees IR and 75 degrees ER. Results show passive joint-position sense in subjects with healthy shoulders improved with brace application. The authors explain the improvement in passive position sense by suggesting a neoprene shoulder brace may stimulate cutaneous mechanoreceptors.

A prospective, randomized study by Walther et al[33] is the only study in the English language to investigate the effectiveness of functional bracing in treating shoulder impingement. Patients diagnosed with outlet impingement were treated using one of the following three methods: conventional physical therapy, a guided self-training program to strengthen the humeral depressors, and a functional brace. Clinical examination, shoulder radiographs, and the Neer test (subacromial injection) determined the diagnosis of impingement. Conventional physical therapy consisted of two to three sessions per week of supervised strengthening exercises and stretching if needed based on initial range of motion measurements. Subjects in the guided self-training group underwent a maximum of four sessions for education on strengthening including elastic resistance exercises for the following muscle groups: humeral head depressors, pectoralis, trapezius, rhomboids, levator scapulae, and serratus anterior. The home program was to be performed five times per week. Subjects in the functional brace group were instructed to wear a Coopercare–Lastrap functional shoulder brace (Coopercare–Lastrap, North York, Ontario, Canada) as long as possible during the day and at night if tolerated. After 12 weeks of treatment, follow-up included assessment of shoulder function using the Constant–Murley score and a pain rating on a visual analog scale. The study found no significant differences with regard to functional improvement or decreased pain between the three treatment groups. The authors suggest improvement of subjects in the functional brace group may be explained by brace influence on proprioception. **Table 8–5** presents a summary of the current research on shoulder braces.

## ◆ Summary

The methods of shoulder taping and bracing described in this chapter may be beneficial due to both mechanical and proprioceptive influences. Although anecdotal evidence reports shoulder taping is effective in decreasing symptoms and improving function, there is no consensus in the scientific research to give these outcomes evidence-based rationale. Shoulder taping may not be effective in limiting ROM, but it may help minimize the risk of injury by increasing proprioception. Further research is needed to determine mechanisms by which tape may be effective at improving shoulder stability and decreasing injury risk. In addition, future research involving pathological shoulders would add to the existing knowledge of shoulder taping effects on normal, healthy shoulders and may provide further evidence for the clinical benefits of shoulder taping in the treatment of orthopedic and neurologic upper-extremity disorders.

Current research does not support brace effectiveness in limiting active or passive ROM to preset brace limits; however, there is some evidence a brace may prevent the shoulder from reaching the vulnerable position of 90 degrees abduction and >90 degrees ER. The numerous types of shoulder braces that exist complicate research on their effectiveness. Further research must be done on the various shoulder braces and their effects on active and passive ROM after sporting activities before definitive conclusions on bracing effects can be made. In addition to motion restriction, the influence of bracing on proprioception and functional performance should be further researched on both healthy and pathological shoulders. The efficacy of shoulder braces in preventing the recurrence of subluxations and dislocations is important to justify their continued use. Regardless of the use or effectiveness of shoulder taping and bracing, the importance of dynamic stability from contractile structures should still be a focus of rehabilitation. Shoulder bracing and taping should be used in addition to appropriate shoulder strengthening exercises discussed in previous chapters.[38-40]

# References

1. Beynnon BD, Good L, Risberg MA. The effect of bracing on proprioception of knees with anterior cruciate ligament injury. J Orthop Sports Phys Ther 2002;32:11–15
2. Cordova ML, Ingersoll CD, LeBlanc MJ. Influence of ankle support on joint range of motion before and after exercise: a meta-analysis. J Orthop Sports Phys Ther 2000;30:170–182
3. Cordova ML, Ingersoll CD, Palmieri RM. Efficacy of prophylactic ankle support: an experimental perspective. J Athl Train 2002;37:446–457
4. Fleming BC, Renstrom PA, Beynnon BD, Engstrom B, Peura G. The influence of functional knee braces on anterior cruciate ligament strain biomechanics in weightbearing and nonweightbearing knees. Am J Sports Med 2000;28:815–824
5. Salsich GB, Brechter JH, Farwell D, Powers CM. The effects of patellar taping on knee kinetics, kinematics, and vastus lateralis muscle activity during stair ambulation in individuals with patellofemoral pain. J Orthop Sports Phys Ther 2002;32:3–10
6. Cools AM, Witvrouw EE, Danneels LA, Cambier DC. Does taping influence electromyographic muscle activity in the scapular rotators in healthy shoulders? Man Ther 2002;7:154–162
7. Morrisey D. Proprioceptive shoulder taping. J Bodywork Mvmt Therapies 2000;4:189–194
8. Alexander CM, Stynes S, Thomas A, Lewis J, Harrison PJ. Does tape facilitate or inhibit the lower fibers of trapezius? Man Ther 2003;8:37–41
9. Hiltbrand J, Running K, Matheson JW, Davies GJ, Kernozek TW. The effects of McConnell taping on shoulder joint position sense. Paper presented at: APTA Annual Conference and Exposition; June 20, 2003; Washington, DC
10. Host HH. Scapular taping in the treatment of anterior shoulder impingement. Phys Ther 1995;75:803–812
11. McConnell J. A novel approach to pain relief pre-therapeutic exercise. J Sci Med Sport 2000;3:325–334
12. Schmitt L, Snyder-Mackler L. Role of scapular stabilizers in etiology and treatment of impingement syndrome. J Orthop Sports Phys Ther 1999;29:31–38
13. Page PA, Stewart GW. Shoulder taping in the management of impingement of the athlete. Med Sci Sports Exerc 1999;31:S208 [ACSM 46th Annual Meeting Abstract]
14. Lewis JS, Wright C, Green A. Subacromial impingement syndrome: the effect of changing posture on shoulder range of movement. J Orthop Sports Phys Ther 2005;35:72–87
15. Kneeshaw D. Shoulder taping in the clinical setting. Journal of Bodywork and Movement Therapies 2002;6:2–8
16. Hamill J, Knutzen KM. Biomechanical Basis of Human Movement. Media, PA: Williams and Wilkins; 1995
17. Coon B, Hart A, Freidhoff C. Case study: tape management of upper extremity reflex sympathetic dystrophy due to chronic shoulder dislocations. J Orthop Sports Phys Ther 1998;27:77 [1998 Combined Sections Meeting Abstract]
18. Peterson C. The use of electrical stimulation and taping to address shoulder subluxation for a patient with central cord syndrome. Phys Ther 2004;84:634–643
19. Shamus JL, Shamus EC. A taping technique for the treatment of acromioclavicular joint sprains: a case study. J Orthop Sports Phys Ther 1997;25:390–394
20. Baquie P. Upper limb taping. Aust Fam Physician 2002; 31:347–349
21. Hanger HC, Whitewood P, Brown G, et al. A randomized controlled trial of strapping to prevent post-stroke shoulder pain. Clin Rehabil 2000;14:370–380
22. Morin L, Bravo G. Strapping the hemiplegic shoulder: a radiographic evaluation of its efficacy to reduce subluxation. Physiother Can 1997;Spring:103–108
23. Mulligan I. Effectiveness of Posterior Shoulder Positioning in Velocity and Isokinetic Shoulder Internal and External Rotation Strength in High School Baseball Pitchers [unpublished doctoral dissertation]. Provo, UT: Rocky Mountain University; 2003
24. Ackermann B, Adams R, Marshall E. The effect of scapula taping on electromyographic activity and musical performance in professional violinists. Aust J Physiother 2002;48:197–203
25. Zanella PW, Willey SM, Seibel SL, Hughes CJ. The effect of scapular taping on shoulder joint repositioning. J Sport Rehabil 2001;10:113–123
26. Morin GE, Tiberio D, Austin G. The effect of upper trapezius taping on electromyographic activity in the upper and middle trapezius region. J Sport Rehabil 1997;6:309–318
27. De Carlo M, Malone K, Gerig J, Hucker M. Evaluation of shoulder instability braces. J Sport Rehabil 1996;5: 143–150
28. Weise K, Sitler MR, Tierney R, Swanik KA. Effectiveness of glenohumeral-joint stability braces in limiting active and passive shoulder range of motion in collegiate football players. J Athl Train 2004;39:151–155
29. Reuss BL, Harding WG III, Nowicki KD. Managing anterior shoulder instability with bracing: an expanded update. Orthopedics 2004;27:614–618
30. Chu JC, Kane EJ, Arnold BL, Gansneder BM. The effect of a neoprene shoulder stabilizer on active joint-reposition sense in subjects with stable and unstable shoulders. J Athl Train 2002;37:141–145
31. DeCarlo M, Malone K. Protective devices for the shoulder complex. In: Hawkins RJ and Misamore GW, eds. Shoulder Injuries in the Athlete: Surgical Repair and Rehabilitation. New York, NY: Churchill Livingstone; 1996:365–373

32. Ulkar B, Kunduracioglu B, Cetin C, Guner RS. The effect of positioning and bracing on passive position sense of shoulder joint. Br J Sports Med 2004;38: 549–552

33. Walther M, Werner A, Stahlschmidt T, Woelfel R, Gohlke F. The subacromial impingement syndrome of the shoulder treated by conventional physiotherapy, self-training, and a shoulder brace: results of a prospective, randomized study. J Shoulder Elbow Surg 2004;13:417–423

34. Marin R. Scapula winger's brace: a case series on the management of long thoracic nerve palsy. Arch Phys Med Rehabil 1998;79:1226–1230

35. Sawa TM. An alternative conservative management of shoulder dislocations and subluxations. J Athl Train 1992;27:366–369

36. McLeod IA, Uhl TL, Arnold BL, Gansneder MN. Effectiveness of shoulder braces in limiting active range of motion [abstract]. J Athl Train 1999;34:S84

37. DeSavage M, Sitler MR, Swanik K. Effects of glenohumeral joint stability braces on restricting active shoulder range of motion during physiological loading [abstract]. J Athl Train 2000;35:S90

38. Moseley JB, Jobe FW, Pink M, Perry J, Tibone J. EMG analysis of the scapular muscles during a shoulder rehabilitation program. Am J Sports Med 1992;20:128–134

39. Reinold MM, Wilk KE, Fleisig GS, et al. Electromyographic analysis of the rotator cuff and deltoid musculature during common shoulder external rotation exercises. J Orthop Sports Phys Ther 2004;34:385–394

40. Townsend H, Jobe FW, Pink M, Perry J. Electromyographic analysis of the glenohumeral muscles during a baseball rehabilitation program. Am J Sports Med 1991;19:264–272

# 9

# Use of Interval Return Programs for Shoulder Rehabilitation

**Todd S. Ellenbecker, Kevin E. Wilk, Michael M. Reinold, Timothy F. Murphy, and Russ Morgan Paine**

In addition to many of the rehabilitation techniques outlined in this text, the formulation of a supervised, progressive program designed to assist patients in their return to full activity is of paramount importance; however, few published reports are available to guide clinicians through this important process. In this chapter, we will provide specific guidelines for the return to sport or interval program for four of the most challenging sport activities for the human shoulder: tennis, baseball, swimming, and golf. In addition to providing the interval program, we will outline some of the unique demands that the glenohumeral joint (GH) undergoes during participation in that sport.

Prior to providing the specific guidelines for each sport, several common characteristics are inherent in each of the four programs detailed in this chapter. First, it is of primary importance that the clinician use specific objectively based guidelines individualized to each patient to determine that patient's readiness to enter an interval sport program. For example, with the exception of golf, all of the sports reviewed in this chapter utilize the 90/90 [90 degrees of abduction and 90 degrees of external rotation (ER)] position as a major force-producing and stabilatory entity. Thus, the patient must demonstrate tolerance to this pattern during resistive exercise and simulated activity prior to actual repetitive sport participation using that position. Tests such as the subluxation relocation maneuver that utilizes the 90-degree abducted position with full ER in an attempt to provoke the GH joint's stabilizing elements including the rotator cuff and labrum can be clinically applied.[1,2] Additionally, muscle performance testing in the 90/90 position is highly recommended to determine the effectiveness of the dynamic stabilizers in functioning in that position. Muscle performance testing can range from simple manual muscle testing to sophisticated isokinetic dynamometry.[3–5]

Second, each of these programs contains a progression from the simplest sport-specific activity to the more challenging. This concept allows for progression of the activity according to the patient's symptoms and recovery status; it enables each program to be tailored specifically to each patient regardless of skill level or degree of involvement in the sport.

Finally, each interval program incorporates proper biomechanical technique to minimize the chance of reinjury and to prevent injury in adjoining segments of the kinetic chain. Of critical importance is the enlistment of an expert who combines extensive training in the biomechanical evaluation of the specific sport with the necessary experience and credential level to initiate actual changes in the patient's biomechanics in relation to the sports activity.

## ◆ The Kinetic Link Principle

The kinetic link principle describes how the human body can be broken down into a series of links or segments, which are interrelated and ultimately affect segments both proximal and distal to that segment. Kibler[6] refers to the kinetic link system as a series of sequentially activated body segments. The kinetic link principle is predicated on a concept developed by Hanavan,[7] who constructed a computerized form of the adult human body composed of conical links connecting the lower extremities, torso, and upper extremities. In upper-extremity skill performance, activity in the upper-extremity segments is transmitted to the trunk and spine via a large musculoskeletal surface. This generates a change of forces across the musculoskeletal surface, which results in the generation of massive amounts of energy.[7]

Davies[8] has described how the upper extremity can be viewed as a series of links. The links proposed by Davies[8] include the trunk, scapulothoracic (ST) articulation, scapulohumeral (SH) or GH joints, and distal arm regions. Each of these links can be independent anatomically and biomechanically, but in relation to human function acts as a unit.

When analyzing human movement, Putnam[9] has discussed the concept of proximal to distal sequencing. This principle states that to produce the largest possible speed at the end of a linked chain of segments, movement must initiate in more proximal segments and proceed to the more distal segment. Additionally, the distal segment motion should commence at the time of maximal speed in the more proximal segment. This concept has been referred to by many names—the *summation of speed principle*,[10] the *kinetic link principle*,[11] and *Palgenhoef's*[12] *concept of acceleration–deceleration.* It has been verified and illustrated by measuring the linear speeds of segment end points, joint angular velocities, as well as joint moments.[13]

Several investigators have reported proximal-to-distal sequencing for kicking a ball, with the hip, knee, and ankle joints reaching their peak speeds in a sequence and each peak being greater than that of the proximal joint.[9] Most researchers feel that the proximal segment deceleration is caused by the acceleration of the distal segment.[9]

Proximal-to-distal sequencing has been reported in the upper extremity during throwing,[14–16] as well as in the tennis serve.[17,18] However, more recent analysis suggests that there are aspects of these upper-extremity patterns (throwing, serving, and striking) that have significant modifications in the traditional proximal-to-distal sequencing. Feltner and Depena[19] reported peak internal rotation (IR) velocity of the humerus following movements of the wrist and hand during overhead throwing, and Sprigings et al[20] have shown IR to be the largest contributor to racquet head velocity at impact despite being one of the last components in the modified sequence of proximal-to-distal sequencing.

Groppel[21] has applied the kinetic link system to the analysis and description of optimal upper-extremity sport biomechanics. Groppel states that the initiation of the sequential activation of the kinetic link system starts at the ground as the lower extremities of the body create a ground reaction force. The sequential activation then proceeds from the legs, through the hips and trunk, and is funneled via the ST and GH joints to the distal aspect of the upper extremity. The important role of both linear and angular momentum in the production of force and power in upper-extremity sport activities such as the throwing motion and tennis serve is clearly evident by analyzing this model. It is important to note that the initiation of movement of the next segment in the kinetic chain occurs prior to complete deceleration of the previous segment. The angular velocity of the segmental rotation in the body's kinetic link system was originally thought to occur at increasingly faster velocities moving from the lower extremities to the upper extremity during the tennis serve.[21] Further biomechanical analysis, however, has

demonstrated that although this sequential increase in angular velocities does occur over many of the segments, a perfect progression in angular velocity does not occur.[17]

Kibler[6] has provided an objective analysis of force generation during a tennis serve. This analysis has identified 54% of the force development during the tennis serve coming from the legs and trunk, with only 25% coming from the elbow and wrist. Nonoptimal performance and increased risk of injury occur in tennis and other sport activities when individuals attempt to utilize the smaller muscles and distal arm segments as a primary source for power generation.[21,22]

## ◆ Tennis

The demands on the GH joint in tennis occur with virtually every ball contact with additional loading occurring during the movements prior to and following ball contact. Electromyographic (EMG) analysis of the tennis serve and groundstrokes finds the highest activity in the rotator cuff muscle tendon unit occurring during the serve.

The tennis serving motion can be broken down into four primary phases: wind-up, cocking, acceleration, and follow-through.[23] These phases are used to scientifically break down the movement and do not occur as separate individual stages or phases during actual performance. Arm cocking occurs as the hands separate and the ball toss is initiated.[23] Dillman et al[24] reported a composite maximal ER angle of the dominant arm of 154 degrees during serving in elite level players. Additionally, during arm cocking when the elbow is in a position of 90 degrees of elbow flexion, dominant arm abduction angles have been reported at 83 degrees in elite Australian players.[17] Inappropriate abduction angles greater than 90 degrees during arm cocking and acceleration may lead to impingement of the rotator cuff tendons under the coracoacromial arch. After maximal external rotation, the dominant shoulder undergoes rapid concentric internal rotation. Angular velocities of 1074 to 1514 deg/s have been measured during the acceleration phase of the tennis serve in elite players.[25] During the acceleration phase, proper evaluation and monitoring are

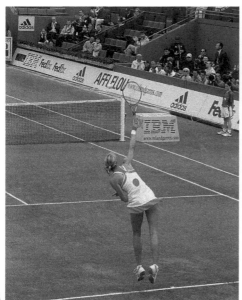
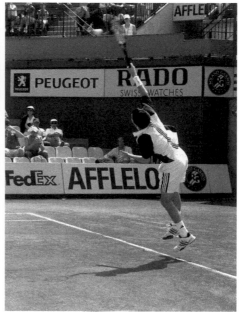

A                                                                                                                                    B

**Figure 9–1**    Tennis serve ball contact illustrating glenohumeral abduction angle between 90 and 100 degrees.

indicated as the hips, trunk, and shoulders segmentally rotate. Premature opening of the hips and trunk can lead to "arm lag" in which the shoulder is placed in extremes of horizontal abduction. This has also been termed *hyperangulation* where the humerus lags behind the scapular plane of the body during IR of the GH joint.[26] This hyperangulation can lead to rotator cuff and labral injury and has been implicated as a major factor in overuse injury in overhead athletes, including tennis players.[26]

For the purpose of analyses, the acceleration phase terminates at ball contact. Initial appearance of GH joint position during ball contact often reveals a nearly vertical humeral position. However, upon closer analysis, the contribution from the trunk via lateral flexion allows the GH joint to be positioned between 90 and 100 degrees (**Fig. 9–1**). This position is critical; it allows for forceful rotational movements with the GH joint below positions with inherent subacromial impingement or compression.[27] Frequently, tennis players with nonoptimal trunk control or stabilization, or players who are unable to laterally flex their trunk to allow for this important alignment use inappropriate amounts of GH abduction during their serve.

Following ball contact, the follow-through phase begins and terminates at the end of the serving motion. The follow-through phase is characterized by significant eccentric muscular activity.[23] A common biomechanical fault found in players with shoulder dysfunction is for the rapid abbreviation of the follow-through phase following ball contact. Recommended technique includes a full motion including trunk flexion and rotation, shoulder extension adduction, and cross-arm adduction as well as IR. Research showing reduced IR range of motion (ROM) in the dominant shoulder of the elite tennis player[28,29] may lead to abbreviated patterns of movement and an increase in scapular upward rotation and protraction. This finding can be compared with the clinical examination findings of total rotation ROM to determine whether abbreviated follow-through patterns are being applied because of a true loss of GH joint IR.

Tennis groundstrokes consist of the forehand and backhand and can be divided into three primary phases: preparation, acceleration, and follow-through. The discrimination between the acceleration and follow-through phases is based upon ball contact. Most consequences for the tennis playing shoulder occur during acceleration and follow-through with the preparation phase showing minimal muscular activity in the shoulder region.[23] One important point regarding the forehand groundstroke preparation phase is the importance of scapular retraction. Placement of the arm behind the body requires horizontal abduction with trunk rotation. Failure to achieve this position with a scapular protracted position may lead to increased anterior shoulder stress particularly as forward trunk rotation is imposed upon this protracted position with the GH joint horizontally abducted.

One very important concept for analysis of the forehand and backhand groundstroke pertains to the position or stance taken by the player during execution. Three primary stances are prevalent: open, square, and closed.[30,31] Traditionally, the square stance has been taught whereby the player stands perpendicular to the net (sideways) with the tips of one foot aligned with the tips of the other foot. The shoulders are also perpendicular to the net and baseline such that upper body and trunk rotation can occur. Players using this type of stance rely primarily on linear momentum to gain power and this is initiated as the player steps forward toward the oncoming ball.[30] Although this classic stance has been used for a very long time, one limitation occurs during follow-through when the pelvis can block further rotation of the trunk and pelvis due to the square stance alignment. This blocking is particularly prevalent when the player uses a truly closed stance where the front foot is placed in a position where it actually crosses over the back foot. This stance is rarely used and not recommended for forehand groundstrokes and would limit the effective transfer of kinetic energy from the lower body and trunk to the upper body for power generation.

The final stance to discuss is the open stance. In today's tennis, nearly all the top players use an open or partially open stance on the forehand with many top players using the open stance for the two-handed backhand as well. The open stance involves placement of the feet parallel to the net or baseline. It is important to note however, that the position of the shoulders must be rotated or closed such that they are placed perpendicular to the pelvis and lower body position and perpendicular to the net or baseline. This allows for greater generation and utilization of angular momentum because of the large angle of separation between the pelvis and shoulders (pelvic/shoulder separation angle). The relationship of the lower extremities in the open stance does not block the pelvis and allows for a more optimal rotation pattern as the upper extremity is accelerated toward the ball and continues through the follow-through phase.[30]

One common error with the open-stance forehand that can lead to anterior shoulder pain and rotator cuff dysfunction occurs during the early rotation of the pelvis when the lower body and trunk rotate ahead of the arm. This improper sequential rotation leaves power generation to the upper body as the trunk and pelvis rotate too early preventing the optimal transfer of power from the lower extremities and trunk. This poorly timed rotation places the GH joint in a position in the coronal plane during ball contact, or in many cases ball contact occurs with even greater amounts of horizontal abduction behind the coronal plane of the body. This creates a position similar to that described during the serving motion of hyperabduction, and when coupled with scapular protraction and imbalanced muscle function can lead to injury or reinjury if these type of mechanics are used in the interval tennis program.[2,27]

The backhand groundstroke can be executed with both one and two hands. Research has shown that muscular activity during the one- and two-handed backhands are statistically similar[31]; however, the use of both hands on the racquet can allow for greater facilitation of trunk rotation and more optimal transfer of energy via the kinetic chain theory. Ball contact should occur slightly in front of the body to allow for a forward progression of the momentum generated. One common error inherent in many players who report pain during the backhand groundstroke is late ball contact. This occurs when the ball is hit while either in line with the body or actually behind the midline (umbilicus) of the body. This results in a nonoptimal transfer of energy from the lower body and trunk and a reliance on concentric shoulder ER for power generation.

Additionally, during the one- and two-handed backhands, the dominant arm is initially brought into some degree of cross-arm adduction during preparation. If the player does not rotate the pelvis and trunk and merely cross-arm adducts (horizontally adducts) the arm, pain may be reported over either the anterior or superior aspect of the shoulder from primary impingement or compression of the rotator cuff under the coracoacromial arch. Careful monitoring of body position and a reliance on rotation of the pelvis and trunk ensure a clear path for arm movement during this important stroke.

## Interval Tennis Program

The specifics of the interval tennis program are outlined in **Table 9–1**. Each of these elements plays an important role in the successful return of the tennis player regardless of skill level. The guidelines for an interval tennis program are presented in **Table 9–2**.

An alternate day format should be followed in the interval program to allow for at least 1 and in some cases 2 days of recovery between sessions. Continuation of the patient's posterior rotator cuff and scapular strengthening program should continue in addition to any formal therapy that is required to normalize ER:IR strength ratios and improve muscular endurance as well as optimize shoulder GH ROM if needed. As mentioned earlier, there is a great emphasis placed on the patient's ability to utilize proper biomechanics. Often when a program is initiated too early because of pressure from the player, coach, or parent, compensatory mechanics are utilized, which may produce injury and introduce inappropriate sport biomechanics. Supervision of the interval program by a certified tennis teaching professional or knowledgeable coach and physical therapist is highly recommended.

The recommended stroke progression is based on the upper-extremity kinetic and kinematic research data that clearly demonstrates significantly lower stress levels on the GH joint during the groundstrokes as compared with the overhead serving motion. The initiation of serving before hitting overhead smashes is also recommended; the serve consists of a self-initiated toss, whereas in the overhead smash the player takes the ball out of the air and must optimally position the shoulder to properly execute the shot.

Preimpact ball velocity is also controlled during the interval tennis program. The ball should be fed by a partner or coach from the net, thus allowing the patient to strike the ball with minimal preimpact ball velocity. This is progressed to having the player rally from the baseline with a partner or coach. Rallying from baseline to baseline produces greater preimpact ball velocities and greater inherent stress to the patient's shoulder during the program.

Further reduction of shoulder stress is achieved by using low-compression or foam tennis balls (EZ Hit Foam Ball, Wilson Sporting Goods, Chicago, IL; low-compression ball or "Star Ball" Penn Racquet Sports, Phoenix, AZ), which are much lighter than the standard tennis ball. These balls when struck by a normal tennis swing go shorter distances, thus facilitating training.

In addition, the type of racquet, string type, and string tension that the player uses should be addressed. Researchers and medical professionals typically recommend racquets that are in the midrange in weight, stiffness, and head size.[32,33] As for string type, "coreless" multifilament strings have been shown to have greater resiliency and thus help protect the arm.

**Table 9–1**    Key Factors in an Interval Tennis Program

| Frequency | Alternate Day Performance |
| --- | --- |
| Supervision | Emphasis on proper stroke mechanics. |
| Stroke pattern progression | Groundstrokes—volleys—serves—overheads progression—matchplay |
| Impact progression | Low preimpact ball velocity to higher preimpact ball velocity |
| Ball progression | Low-compression (foam) to regulation tennis ball |
| Sequencing | Proper warm-up, interval tennis program, cool-down, and cryotherapy |
| Timing | Supplemental rotator cuff and scapular exercises performed either on "rest" day following interval tennis program or after execution of interval tennis program on the same day to minimize the effects of overtraining and overload. |

**Table 9–2**  Interval Tennis Program Guidelines

- Begin at stage indicated by your therapist or doctor.
- Do not progress or continue program if joint pain is present.
- Always stretch your shoulder, elbow, and wrist before and after the interval program, and perform a whole body dynamic warm-up prior to performing the interval tennis program.
- Play on alternate days, giving your body a recovery day between sessions.
- Do not use a wallboard or back board as it leads to exaggerated muscle contraction without rest between strokes.
- Ice your injured arm after each stage of the interval tennis program.
- It is highly recommended to have your stroke mechanics formally evaluated by a USPTA tennis teaching professional.
- Do not attempt to impart heavy topspin or underspin to your groundstrokes until later stages in the interval program.
- Contact your therapist or doctor if you have questions or problems with the interval program.
- Do not continue to play if you encounter localized joint pain.

***Preliminary Stage:***  Foam ball impacts beginning with ball feeds from a partner. Perform 20–25 forehands and backhands assessing initial tolerance to groundstrokes only. Presence of pain or abnormal movement patterns in this stage indicates that you are not ready to progress to the actual interval tennis program. You should continue rehabilitation.

***Interval Tennis Program:***  *Excessive fatigue on your previous outing—Remain at the previous stage or level until you can perform that part of the program without fatigue or pain.*

1.  a.  Have a partner feed 20 forehand groundstrokes to you from the net. (Partner must use a slow, looping feed that results in a waist-high ball bounce for player contact.)
    b.  Have a partner feed 20 backhand groundstrokes as in 1a above.
    c.  Rest 5 minutes.
    d.  Repeat 20 forehand and backhand feeds as above.
2.  a.  Begin as in stage 1 above, with partner feeding 10 forehands and 10 backhands from the net.
    b.  Rally with partner from baseline, hitting controlled groundstrokes until you have hit 50–60 strokes. (Alternate between forehand and backhand and allow 20–30 seconds rest after every 2–3 rallies.)
    c.  Rest 5 minutes.
    d.  Repeat 2b above.
3.  a.  Rally groundstrokes from the baseline for 15 minutes.
    b.  Rest 5 minutes.
    c.  Hit 10 forehand and 10 backhand volleys, emphasizing a contact point in front of body.
    d.  Rally groundstrokes for 15 additional minutes from the baseline.
    e.  Hit 10 forehand and 10 backhand volleys as above.

***Pre-serve Interval:***  (Perform Prior to Stage 4) (Note. This can be performed off court and is meant solely to determine readiness for progression into stage 4 of the interval tennis program.)
    a.  After stretching, with racquet in hand, perform serving motion for 10–15 repetitions without a ball.
    b.  Using a foam ball, hit 10–15 serves without concern for performance result (only focusing on form, contact point, and the presence or absence of symptoms).

4.  a.  Hit 20 minutes of groundstrokes, mixing in volleys using a 70% groundstrokes/30% volleys format.
    b.  Perform 5–10 simulated serves without a ball.
    c.  Perform 5–10 serves using a foam ball.
    d.  Perform 10–15 serves using a standard tennis ball at approximately 75% effort.
    e.  Finish with 5–10 minutes of groundstrokes.
5.  a.  Hit 30 minutes of groundstrokes, mixing in volleys using a 70% groundstrokes/30% volleys format.
    b.  Perform 5–10 serves using a foam ball.
    c.  Perform 10–15 serves using a standard tennis ball at approximately 75% effort.
    d.  Rest 5 minutes
    e.  Perform 10–15 additional serves as in "5c" above.
    f.  Finish with 15–20 minutes of groundstrokes.
6.  a.  Repeat stage 5 listed above increasing the number of serves to 20 to 25 instead of 10 to 15.
    b.  Before resting between serving sessions, have a partner feed easy short lobs to attempt a controlled overhead smash.
7.  Prior to attempting match play, complete steps 1–5 without pain or excess fatigue in the upper extremity. Continue to progress the amount of time rallying with groundstrokes and volleys, in addition to increasing the number of serves per workout until 60–80 overall serves can be performed interspersed throughout a workout. Remember that an average of up to 120 serves can be performed in a tennis match, therefore be prepared to gradually increase the number of serves in the interval program before full competitive play is engaged.

USPTA, United States Professional Tennis Association.

String tension that is overly tight for the racquet frame can increase stress to the extremity of the player; string tensions should be in the midrange of the manufacturer's recommendation. It is beyond the scope of this chapter to cover all aspects of the string and equipment; however, we recommend referring the patient to a USRSA (United States Racquet Stringers Association) certified technician for an evaluation of racquet compatibility and string evaluation.

All of these variables can be manipulated to forward the patient's progression through the interval tennis program. The severity of the injury or surgical procedure should be considered to determine the number of successful trials required at each stage of the interval program. This allows for a controlled progression that can be tailored by the therapist; there can be one trial at each stage of the program or two to three successful trials before progressing to the next level. A *successful* completion implies that the session was performed in a pain-free fashion with no residual postperformance pain. Additionally, the performance of the program did not impair the patient's ability to continue with the rehabilitative exercise program.

## ◆ Baseball

Similar to the demands listed in the previous section for the tennis serve, specific aspects of the throwing motion produce large stresses upon the GH joint; when these stresses are repetitively applied, tissue overload and injury or reinjury can occur.

The baseball pitching motion may be broken down into specific phases, similar to the tennis serve. These phases include the wind-up, stride, arm cocking, arm acceleration, arm deceleration, and follow-through (**Fig. 9–2**). Concerning shoulder pathologies, the arm cocking through arm deceleration phases places the greatest amount of force on the shoulder. Fleisig et al[34] have determined that the greatest amount of kinetic forces at the shoulder occur at the time of maximum ER and ball release.

The cocking phase of the throwing motion occurs following hand separation when the ball leaves the glove and continues until maximal ER of the throwing shoulder occurs.[35] By the end of the cocking phase, the shoulder can obtain a nearly horizontal position of 180 degrees of ER. This amount of ER, however, is combined with ST and trunk articulation and gives the appearance of the artificially high ER value at the shoulder joint.[36] Fleisig et al[34] have suggested that the high amount of forces observed at the GH joint during the cocking phase may lead to pathological anterior glenohumeral hyperlaxity and subsequent rotator cuff and labral lesions associated with internal impingement.

At the time of maximal ER in the throwing arm, it is also important to note that the ST joint must be in a retracted position.[6,26] The scapula actually translates 15 to 18 cm during the throwing motion.[6] Failure to retract the scapula leads to an increase in the antetilting of the glenoid because of a protracted scapular position. This can exacerbate the instability continuum and create anterior instability and suboptimal performance leading to injury.[6,26] Recent research has demonstrated that in late cocking, the abduction and ER position places the posterior band of the inferior GH ligament in a "bowstrung" position under the humeral head. Tightness in this structure can lead to a posterosuperior shift in the humeral head, which can bring on rotator cuff and labral pathology.[26] Improper scapular positioning coupled with increases in horizontal abduction during late cocking and the transition into the acceleration phase has been termed "hyperangulation" and leads to aggravation of undersurface rotator cuff impingement and labral injury derangement.

The acceleration phase begins after maximal ER and ends with the release of the ball. During the delivery phase, the arm initially starts in –30 degrees of horizontal abduction (30 degrees behind the coronal plane).[24] As acceleration of the arm continues, the GH joint is moved forward to a position of +10 degrees of horizontal adduction (10 degrees of horizontal adduction anterior to the coronal plane).[24] During acceleration, the arm moves from a position of 175 to 180 degrees of composite ER to a position of nearly vertical (105) degrees of external rotation at ball release. Internal rotation of the glenohumeral joint during this phase occurs at over 7000 to 9000 deg/s.[24,36]

An additional important variable to monitor during arm cocking and acceleration is the

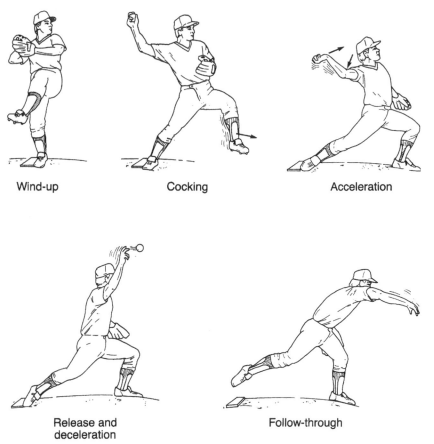

Wind-up      Cocking      Acceleration

Release and
deceleration      Follow-through

**Figure 9–2** Phases of the throwing motion. (From Walsh DA. Shoulder evaluation of the throwing athlete. Sports Med Update 1989;4:24. Also reprinted in Andrews JR, Harrelson GL, Wilk KE. Physical Rehabilitation of the Injured Athlete. 3rd ed. Philadelphia, PA: Saunders; 2004:521, Figure 19–5. Reprinted here by permission)

abduction angle of the GH joint. Research has consistently shown that the abduction angle for the throwing motion ranges between 90 and 110 degrees.[24,37] It is important to note that this angle is relative to the trunk with varying amounts of trunk lateral flexion changing the actual release position while keeping the abduction angle remarkably consistent across individuals and major pitching styles.[24,36,37] Elevation of the GH abduction angle to >110 degrees can subject the rotator cuff to impingement stresses from the overlying acromion. Careful monitoring of this abduction angle during the throwing motion is recommended; still digital images or digital video aids in this regard.

## Interval Baseball Throwing Program

An interval throwing program (ITP) is used to gradually return baseball pitchers and positional players to competition. The ITP is used for high school, collegiate, and professional baseball players and has been developed based on research conducted quantifying the biomechanics of flat-ground, long toss throwing,[38] and partial effort throwing.[39] An athlete can begin an ITP following a satisfactory clinical exam demonstrating full ROM, minimal pain or tenderness, adequate dynamic stabilization, and sufficient strength and muscular endurance.[5,40]

The ITP is set up to minimize the chance of reinjury and emphasizes warm-up and stretching. Because there is an individual variability in all athletes, there is no set timetable for completion of the program. Variability will exist based on the skill level, goals, and injury of each athlete. It is recommended that the athlete follow the program rigidly because this will be the safest route to return to competition. Highly competitive individuals who wish to return to competition quickly have a tendency to increase the intensity of the ITP. This may promote the incidence of reinjury and may retard the rehabilitation process.

The athlete should supplement the ITP with a high-repetition, low-weight exercise program. The strengthening program should achieve a balance between anterior and posterior musculature; however, special emphasis should be given to the posterior rotator cuff and scapular musculature for any strengthening program.[41,42]

The rehabilitation program should follow a sequential order of alternating days.[43] All strengthening, plyometric, and neuromuscular control drills should be performed three times per week (with a day off between days) on the same day as the ITP. The athlete should warm up, stretch, and perform one set of each exercise before the ITP, followed by two sets of each exercise after the ITP. This provides an adequate warm-up but also ensures maintenance of the necessary ROM and flexibility of the upper extremity. Cryotherapy may be used following the completion of a session to

minimize pain and inflammation. The alternate days are used for lower extremity, cardiovascular, and core stability training. In addition, the athlete performs ROM and light strengthening exercises emphasizing the posterior rotator cuff and scapular muscles.[43] The cycle is repeated throughout the week with the seventh day designated for rest and light ROM and stretching exercises (**Table 9–3**).

The ITP is divided into two phases. Phase I is initiated with throwing on flat ground (**Table 9–4**). The athlete begins throwing at 45 feet (13.7 m) and gradually progresses to 60, 90, 120, 150, and 180 feet (18.3, 27.4, 36.6, 45.7, 54.8 m).

A critical aspect of phase I is the use of the "crow-hop" to simulate the throwing act, emphasizing proper body mechanics. Components of the crow-hop method are first a hop, then a skip, followed by the throw. Normally, the velocity of the throw is determined by the distance; however, in the crow-hop, the ball should be thrown with an arc and have only enough momentum to travel the desired distance.

The athlete should begin warm-up throws at a comfortable distance [~30 to 45 feet (9.1 to 13.7 m)] and then progress to the distance indicated for each step of the ITP. The program consists of throwing at each step two to three times on separate days without pain or symptoms before progressing to the next step. Initially, the athlete will perform two sets of 25 throws

**Table 9–3**  Rehabilitation Program for Baseball Players

| Monday | Tuesday | Wednesday | Thursday | Friday | Saturday | Sunday |
|---|---|---|---|---|---|---|
| Throwers 10* | LE strengthening | Throwers 10 | LE strengthening | Throwers 10 | LE strengthening | Light ROM |
| Plyometrics | Cardiovascular | Plyometrics | Cardiovascular | Plyometrics | Cardiovascular | |
| Neuromuscular control drills | Core stability | Neuromuscular control drills | Core stability | Neuromuscular control drills | Core stability | |
| Stretching | Stretching | Stretching | Stretching | Stretching | Stretching | Stretching |
| ITP | Posterior RTC/scapula strengthening** | ITP | Posterior RTC/scapula strengthening* | ITP | Posterior RTC/Scapula strengthening* | |

*Consists of a set of specific exercises designed to increase strength and flexibility of the upper extremity.[4,7]

**Strengthening of the posterior rotator cuff and scapular muscles are incorporated on alternating days during the early phases of rehabilitation. As the overhead athlete progresses to more of a maintenance program, these exercises are discontinued on these days.

ITP, interval throwing program; LE, lower extremity; RTC, rotator cuff; ROM, range of motion.

**Table 9–4**  Interval Throwing Program for Baseball Players: Phase I

| 45' Phase | 60' Phase | 90' Phase | 120' Phase |
|---|---|---|---|
| **Step 1**<br>A. Warm-up throwing<br>B. 45' (25 throws)<br>C. Rest 5–10 minutes<br>D. Warm-up throwing<br>E. 45' (25 throws) | **Step 3**<br>A. Warm-up throwing<br>B. 60' (25 throws)<br>C. Rest 5–10 minutes<br>D. Warm-up throwing<br>E. 60' (25 throws) | **Step 5**<br>A. Warm-up throwing<br>B. 90' (25 throws)<br>C. Rest 5–10 minutes<br>D. Warm-up throwing<br>E. 90' (25 throws) | **Step 7**<br>A. Warm-up throwing<br>B. 120' (25 throws)<br>C. Rest 5-10 min.<br>D. Warm-up throwing<br>E. 120' (25 throws) |
| **Step 2**<br>A. Warm-up throwing<br>B. 45' (25 throws)<br>C. Rest 5–10 minutes<br>D. Warm-up throwing<br>E. 45' (25 throws)<br>F. Rest 5–10 minutes<br>G. Warm-up throwing<br>H. 45' (25 throws) | **Step 4**<br>A. Warm-up throwing<br>B. 60' (25 throws)<br>C. Rest 5–10 minutes<br>D. Warm-up throwing<br>E. 60' (25 throws)<br>F. Rest 5–10 minutes<br>G. Warm-up throwing<br>H. 60' (25 throws) | **Step 6**<br>A. Warm-up throwing<br>B. 90' (25 throws)<br>C. Rest 5–10 minutes<br>D. Warm-up throwing<br>E. 90' (25 throws)<br>F. Rest 5–10 minutes<br>G. Warm-up throwing<br>H. 90' (25 throws) | **Step 8**<br>A. Warm-up throwing<br>B. 120' (25 throws)<br>C. Rest 5-10 min.<br>D. Warm-up throwing<br>E. 120' (25 throws)<br>F. Rest 5-10 min.<br>G. Warm-up throwing<br>H. 120' (25 throws)<br>(Pitchers go to step 14) |

| 150' Phase | 180' Phase |
|---|---|
| **Step 9**<br>A. Warm-up throwing<br>B. 150' (25 throws)<br>C. Rest 5–10 minutes<br>D. Warm-up throwing<br>E. 150' (25 throws) | **Step 11**<br>A. Warm-up throwing<br>B. 180' (25 throws)<br>C. Rest 5–10 minutes<br>D. Warm-up throwing<br>E. 180' (25 throws) |
| **Step 10**<br>A. Warm-up throwing<br>B. 150' (25 throws)<br>C. Rest 5–10 minutes<br>D. Warm-up throwing<br>E. 150' (25 throws)<br>F. Rest 5–10 minutes<br>G. Warm-up throwing<br>H. 150' (25 throws) | **Step 12**<br>A. Warm-up throwing<br>B. 180' (25 throws)<br>C. Rest 5–10 minutes<br>D. Warm-up throwing<br>E. 180' (25 throws)<br>F. Rest 5–10 minutes<br>G. Warm-up throwing<br>H. 180' (20 throws) |
| | **Step 13**<br>A. Warm-up throwing<br>B. 180' (25 throws)<br>C. Rest 5–10 minutes<br>D. Warm-up throwing<br>E. 180' (25 throws)<br>F. Rest 5–10 minutes<br>G. Warm-up throwing<br>H. 180' (25 throws) 120 → 90'<br>I. Rest 5–10 minutes<br>J. Warm-up throwing<br>K. 15 throws |
| | **Step 14:** Return to respective position or progress to step 14 below. |

All throws should be on an arc with a crow-hop Warm-up throws consist of 10–20 throws at approximately 30 feet Throwing program should be performed every other day, 3 times per week unless otherwise specified by your physician or rehabilitation specialist. Perform each step 2–3 times before progressing to next step.

**Flat-Ground Throwing for Baseball Pitchers**

**Step 14**
A. Warm-up throwing
B. Throw 60 ft. (10–15 throws)
C. Throw 90 ft. (10 throws)
D. Throw 120 ft. (10 throws)
E. Throw 60 ft. (flat ground) using pitching mechanics (20–30 throws)

**Step 15**
A. Warm-up throwing
B. Throw 60 ft. (10–15 throws)
C. Throw 90 ft. (10 throws)
D. Throw 120 ft. (10 throws)
E. Throw 60 ft. (flat ground) using pitching mechanics (20–30 throws)
F. Throw 60-90 ft. (10–15 throws)
G. Throw 60 ft. (flat ground) using pitching mechanics (20 throws)

Progress to Phase II, Throwing Off the Mound

*Note:* 45 feet = 13.7 meters; 60 feet = 18.3 meters; 90 feet = 27.4 meters; 120 feet = 36.6 meters; 150 feet = 45.7 meters; 180 feet = 54.8 meters.

at the specified distance. Adequate warm-up before each set and a rest of 5 to 10 minutes are encouraged. The amount of throws is then increased to three sets of 25 throws at each distance and finally to the next distance in the sequence. If pain or symptoms arise at a particular step, the athlete is instructed to return to the previous asymptomatic step and attempt to progress again when symptoms subside.

Positional players are instructed to progress through the entire ITP before beginning position-specific drills. However, pitchers are instructed to progress through 120 feet (36.6 m) of long toss throwing (step 8 of phase I). At this time, they may opt to continue the normal progression or they may advance to step 14 of phase I. This step is intended specifically for pitchers and involves 10 to 15 throws at progressive distances of 60, 90, and 120 feet (18.3, 27.4, and 36.6 m), followed by flat-ground throwing from 60 feet (18.3 m) using their normal pitching mechanics. This is the first time pitchers are allowed to throw in a straight line without a crow-hop and an arc in the throw.

After the pitcher can perform phase I without symptoms they will be ready to progress to phase II, throwing off a mound (**Table 9–5**). Just as the advancement to this point has been gradual and progressive, the return to unrestricted pitching must follow the same principles. The length of phase II is determined specifically for each athlete. A pitcher should first throw only fastballs at a 50% level of effort, progressing to 75 and 100% levels. The level of effort is often difficult for the athlete to perceive. Fleisig et al[39] have determined that when athletes are instructed to throw at their 75% level of effort, the ball's actual velocity was measured at their 90% level. Similarly, when asked to throw at a 50% level, the actual ball velocity was 85% of their full throwing speed. The use of a radar gun is a helpful tool in effort control.

Phase II of the ITP begins by using the 120 feet (36.6 m) step of phase I as a warm-up. The pitcher then throws 15 throws off the mound using full wind-up pitching mechanics at a 50% level of effort. As the player progresses through phase II, the number of pitches as well as the throwing level of effort is gradually advanced until the athlete is allowed to pitch at light batting practice. At this time, the player may start more stressful pitches such as breaking balls as well as the initiation of simulated games.

During the recovery process, the athlete may experience soreness and a dull, diffuse aching sensation in the muscles and tendons. If sharp pain is felt, particularly in the joint or point of injury, the athlete is instructed to stop all sport activity until the pain ceases. If pain persists, the athlete needs to undergo a physical assessment.

Furthermore, the use of proper throwing mechanics is critical during the ITP. It is imperative that the athlete minimize mechanical faults that may increase stress on the throwing shoulder and elbow such as leading with the elbow, dropping the elbow, and closing the stance during foot contact. A pitching coach or someone proficient in sports biomechanics is a valuable ally to the rehabilitation team to ensure that proper throwing mechanics are used.

An ITP for Little League–aged athletes may also be applied. The Little League ITP (**Table 9–6**) parallels the previously outlined ITP in providing the young baseball player with a graduated progression of throwing distances. Alterations are made based on the size of Little League fields and the distance from home plate to the mound compared with high school and adult playing situations. Similar warm-up and flexibility exercises are incorporated. The Little League player begins throwing with a warm-up consisting of lobbing the ball 15 to 20 feet (4.6 to 6.1 m). The player then performs two sets of 25 throws at 30 feet (9.1 m) with a 15-minute rest in between. As the athlete progresses, three sets of 25 throws are initiated. The Little League player is progressed from 30 feet to 45, 60, and 90 feet (9.1 m to 13.7, 18.3, and 27.4 m) followed by positional drills and pitching off the mound similar to phase II of the ITP.

## ◆ Swimming

Unlike the highly structured interval return progressions associated with sports whose mechanisms are based upon a return from a period of little or no activity, plans for returning the swimmer to unrestricted training and competition are fraught with variables, which are as unique as the athletes themselves. Depending on the nature and degree of their injury, swimmers may be returning to training

**Table 9–5** Interval Throwing Program for Baseball Players: Phase II, Throwing Off the Mound*

| Stage One: Fastballs Only | All throwing off the mound should be done in the presence of your pitching coach or sport biomechanist to stress proper throwing mechanics |
|---|---|
| **Step 1: Interval throwing**<br>15 Throws off mound 50% | |
| **Step 2: Interval throwing**<br>30 Throws off mound 50% | *(Use speed gun to aid in effort-level control)* |
| **Step 3: Interval throwing**<br>45 Throws off mound 50% | *Use interval throwing 120 ft (36.6m) phase as warm-up* |
| **Step 4: Interval throwing**<br>60 Throws off mound 50% | |
| **Step 5: Interval throwing**<br>70 Throws off mound 50% | |
| **Step 6: 45 throws off mound 50%**<br>30 Throws off mound 75% | |
| **Step 7: 30 throws off mound 50%**<br>45 Throws off mound 75% | |
| **Step 8: 10 throws off mound 50%**<br>65 Throws off mound 75% | |
| **Stage Two: Fastballs only** | |
| **Step 9: 60 throws off mound 75%**<br>15 Throws in batting practice | |
| **Step 10: 50–60 throws off mound 75%**<br>30 Throws in batting practice | |
| **Step 11: 45–50 throws off mound 75%**<br>45 Throws in batting practice | |
| **Stage Three**<br>**Step 12: 30 throws off mound 75% warm-up**<br>15 Throws off mound 50% Begin breaking balls<br>45–60 Throws in batting practice (fastball only) | |
| **Step 13: 30 throws off mound 75%**<br>30 Breaking balls 75%<br>30 Throws in batting practice | |
| **Step 14: 30 throws off mound 75%**<br>60-90 Throws in batting practice Gradually increase breaking balls | |
| **Step 15: Simulated game: progressing by 15 throws per workout (pitch count)** | |

*Level of effort = %.

from scratch, from a break of several days to weeks, or from a temporary reduction in training intensity.

## Injuries in Swimmers

The majority of the musculoskeletal problems facing the competitive swimmer are seen at the shoulder, with up to 73% of swimmers at the elite and collegiate levels experiencing shoulder pain that limits training at some point in their career.[44–47] A significant volume of overuse injuries are prevalent in this sport, based primarily on the high volume of repetitive overhead movements.

The classic symptom complex associated with swimmers' shoulder pain involves subacromial impingement. In most cases, this is related to fatigue-related changes in stroke mechanics in individuals with GH hypermobility or instability. In a small number of swimmers, impingement is related to hypomobility and inflexibility, particularly with limitations in scapular retraction and upward rotation leading to increased

15

**Table 9–6** Little League Interval Throwing Program

| 30' Phase | 45' Phase |
|---|---|
| **Step 1** | **Step 3** |
| A. Warm-up throwing | A. Warm-up throwing |
| B. 30' (25 throws) | B. 45' (25 throws) |
| C. Rest 15 minutes | C. Rest 15 minutes |
| D. Warm-up throwing | D. Warm-up throwing |
| E. 30' (25 throws) | E. 45' (25 throws) |
| | |
| **Step 2** | **Step 4** |
| A. Warm-up throwing | A. Warm-up throwing |
| B. 30' (25 throws) | B. 45' (25 throws) |
| C. Rest 10 minutes | C. Rest 10 minutes |
| D. Warm-up throwing | D. Warm-up throwing |
| E. 30' (25 throws) | E. 45' (25 throws) |
| F. Rest 10 min. | F. Rest 10 minutes |
| G. Warm-up throwing | G. Warm-up throwing |
| H. 30' (25 throws) | H. 45' (25 throws) |

| 60' Phase | 90' Phase |
|---|---|
| **Step 5** | **Step 7** |
| A. Warm-up throwing | A. Warm-up throwing |
| B. 60' (25 throws) | B. 90' (25 throws) |
| C. Rest 15 minutes | C. Rest 15 minutes |
| D. Warm-up throwing | D. Warm-up throwing |
| E. 60' (25 throws) | E. 90' (25 throws) |
| | |
| **Step 6** | **Step 8** |
| A. Warm-up throwing | A. Warm-up throwing |
| B. 60' (25 throws) | B. 90' (20 throws) |
| C. Rest 10 min. | C. Rest 10 min. |
| D. Warm-up throwing | D. Warm-up throwing |
| E. 60' (25 throws) | E. 60' (20 throws) |
| F. Rest 10 minutes | F. Rest 10 minutes |
| G. Warm-up throwing | G. Warm-up throwing |
| H. 60' (25 throws) | H. 45' (20 throws) |
| | I. Rest 10 minutes |
| | J. Warm-up throwing |
| | K. 45' (15 throws) |

*Note:* 30 feet = 9.1 meters; 45 feet = 13.7 meters; 60 feet = 18.3 meters; 90 feet = 27.4 meters.

subacromial compressive loads.[48] These restrictions can also be factors in the development of upper-quarter neurovascular symptoms. Additionally, swimmers present with a variety of muscular irritation and tendinitis, particularly in the biceps (long and short heads), posterior rotator cuff, and periscapular muscles.

## Training Stresses in Swimmers

At the competitive age group and high school levels, the frequency of overhead cycles exceeds any other overhead sporting activity, and at the elite level, the number of end-range overhead movements is staggering. Based on a conservative estimate of 8 stroke cycles per 25 yards, a swimmer performing a 10,000 yard workout may expect to complete as many as 3200 overhead cycles with each arm during the workout. In some extreme cases, a swimmer may reach overhead as many as 2 million times over the course of a year.[49]

Interestingly, as swimmers fatigue and begin to experience a breakdown in stroke mechanics, they lose efficiency and take more strokes to complete a given distance, compounding the abnormal biomechanical forces leading to their pathology. Without question, fatigue is the leading factor to stroke breakdown and the onset of symptoms. The majority of swimmers experience no symptoms until they are well into their workout, or when they are performing particularly fatiguing activity (sprint sets, long-distance intervals). Swimmers, in the course of developing overuse problems, relate gradual onset of symptoms late in their workout. As the irritation progresses and performance degrades, the onset of symptoms occurs progressively earlier in the swim. The temporal onset of symptoms in swim training forms the basis for much of the strategy involved in returning the injured swimmer to fully functional training levels.

Typical swim training is really a form of "controlled" overtraining. Swimmers push training to the extent that their performance is actually degraded to the point that midseason performances are rarely record efforts. When training is "tapered" at some strategic point (usually just several weeks before key championships), there is a resultant surge in performance and significant drop in race times.[50-53]

Up to 60 to 80% of swim workouts involve freestyle swimming, regardless of stroke or event specialty.[50-53] For that reason, most swimmers may be evaluated based on symptom presentation in freestyle swimming. Freestyle is also the preferred stroke "vehicle" by which swim training is progressed (**Fig. 9–3**). Unlike the butterfly stroke, and to a lesser extent, the backstroke, body roll may be exaggerated in freestyle to relieve shoulder stress, and the overhead stroke reach may be reduced to avoid shoulder stress. The ultimate goal is to achieve unrestricted performance of

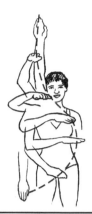

**Figure 9–3** Phases of the freestyle stroke. (From Cousilman JE. The Science of Swimming. Englewood Cliffs, NJ: Prentice Hall; 1968. Also reprinted in Page P, Ellenbecker T. The Scientific and Clinical Application of Elastic Resistance. Champaign, IL: Human Kinetics; 2003, Figure 18.05, p. 239. Reprinted here by permission.)

the desired stroke without compensation, but the interval progression may involve the "buying" of extra yards at the expense of technique as a legitimate tool in tolerating the overhead stresses of this sport.

## Interval Programs for Swimmers

The individual nature of swim training based upon stroke and competitive distance, training patterns, age, and competitive level as well as differences in coaching philosophy, virtually guarantees the need for the development of a unique return plan for each and every swimmer encountered by the health care professional. It is unlikely that the swimmer will successfully complete a progression to unrestricted training if they have not been able to demonstrate good progress in symptomatic management and the achievement of the fundamental capabilities of performing the swimming stroke.[54] Key criteria for implementation of a transitional swimming program include:

- Full ROM, including adequate upward scapular rotation to allow for appropriate streamline position (full flexion/abduction) without impingement
- Pain-free tolerance of rotator cuff and scapular strengthening routines, including

resisted movement into provocative overhead positions
- Ability to perform a swim of at least 500 yards at warm-up intensity (50% of normal training intensity level) without symptoms

Injury scenarios involving the need for a structured swimming progression fall into several typical patterns. Understanding the factors leading to pathology, as well as the timeframe for appropriate recovery, guides the progression of training.[44,45,54,55] Several key scenarios and their specific interval progression elements are listed here.

### In-Season Management of Training Errors or Progressive Overuse

The swimmer's history of symptoms will frequently indicate an onset associated with a training error (too far, too fast, too soon) involving some significant change in training intensity, such as a rapid progression at the onset of the training season, a midseason surge in training (holiday break), or increased stresses through the introduction of exaggerated drills. Many times the swimmer experiences symptoms several weeks after the change, clouding the source of the pathology. In these situations, appropriate management starts with the reduction of training to subclinical levels,[55,56] and the subsequent reprogression of swim training using interval progression methods. Usually, the athlete notices initial onset of symptoms either after or at the end of their workout. Over time, the symptoms occur earlier and earlier in the workout as fatigue-related changes in technique accompany progressive muscular weakness.

- Identify onset of symptoms in workout.
- Reduce training to some level (~500 yards) below symptom threshold (i.e., if swimmer notes onset of symptoms 2500 yards into the workout, reduce training to 2000 as a starting point).
- Initiate remedial rotator cuff and scapular stabilization exercise.
- Begin progression of training distance as exercise tolerance allows athlete to exercise with intensity—usually this can begin within 1 week.
- Identify training distance goal and timeframe for progression.

- The swimmer should be able to complete 3000 yards at warm-up intensity before implementing intervals or send-offs.
- Be careful not to add distance and intensity at the same time. A more conservative progression might be to add intensity on prime days and distance on off days.

## Return to Swimming after Termination of Training

Occasionally, swimmers will need to be reintroduced to training after complete cessation of swimming, such as a return after surgery, an acute episode of instability, or a "runaway" progression of inflammatory symptoms to the point at which training must be terminated.[54-58] Situations involving the complete cessation of swimming activities are relatively rare; however, significant injury or surgery must involve total rest from overhead activity. This type of situation involves a more careful and conservative return strategy, potentially over a period of months rather than weeks.

- Begin swims after ROM is complete and adequate for overhead repetitions (swimming should not be used as a tool to regain range), and appropriate strengthening activities are tolerated without symptoms.
- Keep frequency to three/week for the first 2 to 4 weeks.
- Begin easy off days after 2 to 4 weeks.
- Equalize daily training after 2 to 4 weeks of beginning off-day training.
- Establish goals for attainment of unrestricted levels based on the tolerance of initial swims and the magnitude of the problem (injury/surgery) that precipitated the break from training.
- Initial progression should be no more than 10% per week; however, the rate of progression may increase with time based on tolerance.
- The coach should be involved in the progression of training intensity once initial tolerance is established and base-level training is achieved.

## Off-Season Progression of Training

Many swimmers wait for the termination of the competitive season, accepting their symptoms in lieu of a therapeutic alteration of training rather than risking a failure of their taper.[55,56] The off-season usually allows adequate time for a more gradual progression of distance and intensity (10% or less of base per week). The swimmer may be more likely to take a brief break from intense swim training, allowing for the implementation of focused, remedial training on land, interspersed with controlled swims of reduced intensity and frequency. For year-round competitive swimmers, this break may be only a few weeks in duration; for many others there is a noncompetitive period of several months.

- If possible, allow the swimmer to take a break from swim training for 2 to 4 weeks, concentrating on symptom reduction and remedial strengthening.
- Reintroduce swim training at warm-up intensity at no more than 50% of the eventual training goal.
- Determine weekly training frequency. Three swims per week may work well for noncompetitive periods, but training should be ramped-up so that the swimmer can be comfortable with daily, intense training leading into the next competitive cycle.

## General Strategies for All Swim Progression Programs

Once daily training begins, take advantage of easy days (lighter training days on Tuesdays/Thursdays) for the initial 50 to 70% of the progression.

- As with all interval sports progressions, drop back to the last successfully completed level if symptoms are encountered.
- Build in plateau points as frequently as needed (weekly, bimonthly, etc.) to make sure that the swimmer is tolerating progressions without some looming increase in symptoms.
- There are several methods to divide training progression based on the perceived tolerance of the swimmer for increases.
  - Divide increase goal by available time to get steps leading to a daily increase in training (i.e., increase 200 yards per day).

- Jump training by weekly yardage totals (i.e., 1 week at 500 yards followed by 1 week at 1000 yards).
- Progression recommendations are something best determined by experience. Generally, swimming distance is not progressed faster than 15 to 30% of the base per week (i.e., at a base of 3000 yards, do not progress more than 500 to 1000 yards on a weekly basis).
- Swimmers should be able to tolerate a warm-up pace training level (~50% normal intensity) equivalent to 40 to 60% of their distance goal prior to incorporating increases in intensity, so if the training goal is 6000 yards per day, make sure the swimmer can handle 3000 yards or more per day of warm-up intensity before beginning intervals, send-offs, etc.).
- Avoid any sudden increases in training distance or intensity. Holiday break (no school/no meets) is a notorious time for drastically increasing training; an injured swimmer should be closely supervised during this time.
- Avoid any new or exaggerated training drills that may place additional stress on the injury. One common drill (the zipper drill) involves bringing the thumb to the armpit during recovery before completing the stroke as a method of encouraging high elbow recovery. This drill actually reproduces the impingement sign with every overhead movement—usually with predictable increases in symptoms for the injured swimmer.
- If any strokes are pain-free, incorporate a shift in emphasis to the nonoffending stroke for a kind of in-pool cross-training.
- Incorporate frequent breaks in the workout to reduce fatigue-related stroke breakdown.
- Use observation and/or feedback from the swimmer regarding their experience with stroke breakdown—the workout set should be terminated at the first sign of fatigue-related stroke degradation.
- Once initial base is achieved, further progression of distance and pace should be determined with the assistance of the coach.
- Divide warm-up pace training into sets of tolerable distances (i.e., 500 yards). Increase the number of sets initially, then the duration (distance) of sets as fatigue-resistance develops,
- Flexibility restrictions are rarely the primary problem in swimmers' injuries, but if they are, frequent breaks for stretching are indicated.
- The use of fins or "zoomers" (1/2 fins) may allow the swimmer to reduce shoulder stress associated with primary propulsion, and allow for a greater number of pain-free overhead cycles.
- To accommodate an interval swimming progression, the swimmer should be prepared for several extra steps in the performance of their daily training routine.
- Practice pattern

1. Warm-up—general stretches
2. Specific flexibility exercises (if indicated)
3. Light warm-up exercises (cords)
4. Warm-up swim
5. Rest interval
6. Repeat stretches (if indicated)
7. Modified training set
8. Repeat steps 5 to 7 according to established plan
9. Repeat stretches (if indicated)
10. Ice

Implementation of interval sports progression for the competitive swimmer is a process that involves a healthy dose of common sense combined with fundamental clinical management. It cannot be accomplished without first gaining the confidence of the swimmer. The progression must make sense not only to the clinician and the swimmer, but to the parent and the coach as well. The key element in this process is the strategic management of fatigue because this component alone is the most significant factor in the onset of symptoms in the swimmer. The goal of management is to push the fatigue point later and later into the workout, until it is no longer encountered as a limiting factor. A properly implemented training progression can lead to the successful completion of the competitive season by athletes who would otherwise be lost to training interruptions or termination due to pain and dysfunction.

## ◆ Golf

The game of golf is becoming more and more popular as a spectator and participant sport; it is one of the top recreational activities in our country today. Over 24 million Americans currently play golf and another 2 million are beginning to play each year. To the nonplayer, golf is often considered a leisure game. However, as we all know, golf is a sport that requires athletic skills such as strength, power, flexibility, and coordination to swing a golf club over 100 miles per hour and hit the ball over 200 yards.[59]

Although not viewed as a vigorous sport, golf cannot be considered a benign activity. Studies have revealed that golf injuries occur in 62% of those individuals who play golf.[60] In a survey of the injury rates of men and women professional golfers, it was concluded that the highest incidence of injury was to the left wrist (23.9%), followed by the back (23.7%), left hand (7.1%), and left shoulder (6.9%).[61] In a similar study among amateur players, the back was the most commonly injured (24.2%), followed by the elbow (23.2%), the hand and the wrist (14.1%), and the shoulder (8.3%).[62]

The most common cause of injuries to the golfer is repetitive overuse from both practicing and playing. In an epidemiological study, Gosheger et al[63] determined that 82.6% of injuries were attributed to overuse. Poor physical conditioning, abnormal posture control, and faulty swing mechanics also contribute to golf injuries.

### Electromyographic Analysis of the Golf Swing

To isolate and identify the functions of the major muscles controlling the various body segments during the golf swing, dynamic electromyographic (EMG) and high-speed motion analysis are frequently utilized. The phases of the golf swing and the EMG recording are synchronized to study specific muscle firing patterns at defined moments in the golf swing. Through these investigations, objective evidence is provided for rehabilitative and preventative exercises, training and conditioning, and surgical procedures for the golfer.

For discussion and analysis purposes, the golf swing has been broken down into the following five phases (**Fig. 9–4**):[64]

1. Takeaway: From address the ball to the end of the backswing
2. Forward swing: From the end of the backswing until the club is horizontal
3. Acceleration: From horizontal position of the club to ball contact
4. Early follow-through: From ball contact to horizontal club position
5. Late follow-through: From horizontal club position to the end of the swing

### Takeaway

Before initiation of the backswing, the golfer must have the proper setup and ball address. This initial posture greatly influences the balance of forces throughout the golf swing and is therefore critical to the achievement of the proper swing plane. The takeaway phase has been described as a *coiling* or *loading* of the body to enhance the velocity and kinetic energy of the clubhead.[65]

An EMG analysis reveals relatively low activity of the trunk musculature during this segment of the golf swing because the trunk is simply preparing for the swing.[64] An EMG analysis of the scapular muscles of the trailing arm reveals relatively high activity of the upper, middle, and lower portions of the trapezius during takeaway to help the scapula retract and upwardly rotate.[66] Similarly, the levator scapulae and rhomboid muscle of the trailing arm are active during this period to help with such scapular movements.[66] In the leading arm during takeaway, the activity of the scapular stabilizing muscles is relatively low to allow for scapular protraction.

An EMG analysis of the rotator cuff muscles exhibits contributions from the supraspinatus and infraspinatus in the trailing arm as they act to approximate and stabilize the shoulder.[65,67] Of the rotator cuff muscles in the leading arm, only the subscapularis was shown to display marked activity in the takeaway phase. An EMG analysis also reveals activity of the common wrist extensor muscles during this segment of the golf swing.[68] The pectoralis major, the latissimus dorsi, and the deltoid muscles of both arms are relatively inactive in the golfer's backswing of the golf club.[65,67]

### Forward Swing

During forward swing, trunk rotation movement is initiated. Pink et al[64] demonstrated backside erector spinae and bilateral abdominal oblique muscle activation to counteract the downward movement of the trunk.[64]

Analysis of the trailing arm scapular muscles shows that the three portions of the trapezius taper to allow for scapular protraction.[66] However, the levator scapula and rhomboid muscles display marked activity to control scapular protraction and rotation of the trailing

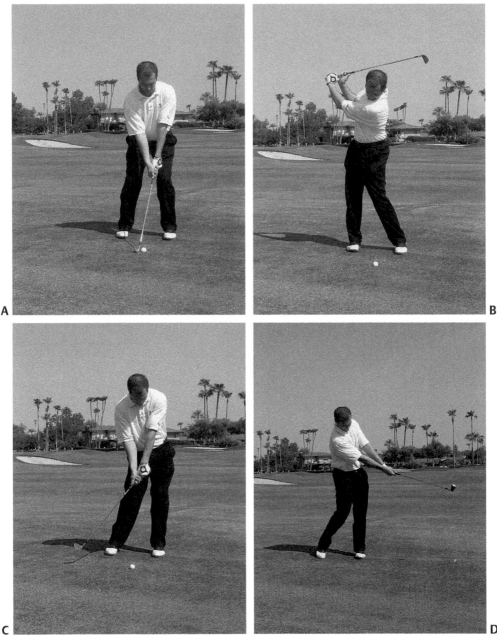

**A**

**B**

**C**

**D**

**Figure 9–4** Phases of the Golf Swing. **(A)** Golf address. **(B)** Golf takeaway. **(C)** Golf acceleration. **(D)** Early follow-through. (*Continued on page 158*)

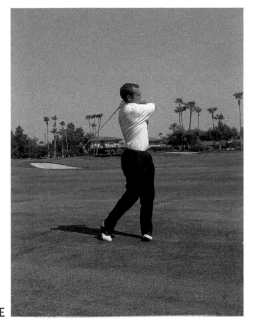

**E**

**Figure 9–4** (*Continued*)   Phases of the Golf Swing. **(E)** Late follow-through.

arm. Analysis of the serratus anterior muscle in the trailing show increased activity during forward swing to aid in scapular protraction.[66] EMG studies of the lead arm demonstrate high activity of the trapezius, levator scapulae, rhomboid, and serratus anterior muscles as they all contribute to scapular motion and stabilization as the arms move toward the ball.[66]

Of the trailing shoulder muscles during forward swing, the subscapularis, pectoralis major, and latissimus dorsi muscles begin firing at marked levels as the trailing arm increasingly accelerates into the IR and adduction. The lead arm subscapularis and latissimus dorsi are both moderately active during the forward swing phase.

### Acceleration

In the acceleration phase, the body segments work together in a coordinated sequence to maximize clubhead speed at ball impact. During this phase, there are consistent EMG levels of the erector spinae and abdominal oblique muscle bilaterally. Peak activity of the lead side erector spinae is seen at this time. The erector spinae are continuing to control the forward fall of the trunk while the oblique

muscles are responsible for rotation of the trunk.[64]

Only the serratus anterior is active in the trailing arm scapular muscles during acceleration.[66] The serratus anterior muscle allows for a strong scapular protraction and contributes to maximizing clubhead speed. Conversely, an EMG analysis reveals strong contractions of the scapular muscles in the lead arm during acceleration.[66] The trapezius, levator scapula, and rhomboid muscles are firing to aid in scapular retraction, upward rotation, and elevation. The serratus anterior muscle of the lead arm continues to display activation.

High subscapularis, pectoralis major, and latissimus dorsi contractions provide power to the trailing arm during the acceleration swing segment as shown on EMG.[67] These muscles further increase in activity from forward swing to assist in rotation and forceful adduction of the arm. The latissimus dorsi muscle contributes the most power in the forward swing, whereas the pectoralis major muscle supplies the most power during acceleration.[65] Likewise, the subscapularis, pectoralis major, and latissimus dorsi muscles of the lead arm fire at high rates during the acceleration swing phase.[65,67] The common wrist flexor muscles of the trail arm produce a sudden burst of activity at ball contact.[68]

### Early Follow-Through

After ball contact has been made, the follow-through phase is initiated. During early follow-through, the body segments now work to decelerate their rotatory contributions, often through eccentric muscle contractions.[64,67] Trunk muscle activity during follow-through, although of low intensity, remains consistent to aid in proper postural control and energy dissipation.[64]

The scapular muscles of the trailing arm display decreased activity throughout the follow-through phases, allowing for coordinated scapular protraction.[66] Likewise, the scapular muscles of the lead arm display tapered activity through these swing segments. The serratus anterior muscles of both arms show consistent muscle firing patterns through the follow-through phases.[66]

In the trailing shoulder, marked activity of the subscapularis, pectoralis major, and latissimus dorsi muscles persisted into the early follow-through.[67] For the lead shoulder, only the subscapularis muscle continued its level of activity, while the pectoralis major and latissimus dorsi muscles decreased their contributions.[65,67]

*Late Follow-Through*

As the golfer finishes the swing, muscle activity of the trunk remains relatively low.[64] Activity of the scapular muscle of both arms taper to low levels as the swing comes to an end.[66] Only the subscapularis muscle of the trailing shoulder remained highly active during this phase.[65,67] Bilaterally, the pectoralis major and latissimus dorsi muscles continue to fire at decreasing levels. Analysis of the lead arm reveals marked activity of the infraspinatus and the supraspinatus rotator cuff muscles.[65] The common wrist extensor muscles fire at low levels, acting to decelerate wrist flexion during this terminal phase of the golf swing.[68]

## Pathomechanical Analysis of the Golf Swing

Although it is not our goal here to describe the proper mechanics of the golf swing, common swing faults and mechanical deficiencies will be described to allow for a better understanding of the proper strengthening, conditioning, and flexibility principles that follow. In addition, recommended alterations in the golf swing will be given for those who may need to compensate for current or chronic orthopedic issues.

Before analyzing the golf swing, the setup posture and address should be examined. The most common mistake seen at setup is the use of spinal flexion by the golfer to position over the ball rather than utilizing a hip-hinge motion.[60] When this spinal flexion is maintained, the golfer's center of gravity will remain posterior to the base of support. This posture will, in turn, place additional loads through the spine and will increase the stresses placed upon the spinal structures throughout the swing.[60]

To maintain proper spine angles, utilize proper rotation, and achieve balance throughout the golf swing, the golfer needs excellent hip, shoulder, and trunk flexibility. Limitations in flexibility will cause the golfer to sacrifice

essential fundamentals and place undue stresses on the lower back during the golf swing.[60] For example, a golfer with limited trunk flexibility will compensate by producing more rotation in the lumbar spine and pelvic girdle. This will place increased stresses on hypomobile or hypermobile spinal segments. Furthermore, instructors often recommend restricted hip turn with increased trunk and shoulder rotation. This is to increase swing power and distance. However, this may be at the expense of increased low back problems.

During takeaway, the lead arm is placed into increasing degrees on internal rotation and cross-body adduction. This position may predispose the golfer to impingement type problems as the rotator cuff tendons and bursae are compressed within the shoulder.[69] At the end of the backswing, forces on the acromioclavicular (AC) joint of the lead arm are shown to be high, contributing to the incidence of pain seen in the golfer's shoulder.

The posterior rotator cuff and scapular muscles of the lead arm are also placed at risk for injury at the top of the backswing as they are placed under a stretch-load.[70] Kao et al[66] commented that the levator scapulae and rhomboid muscles are often injured in this end-range position.

During forward swing and acceleration, high muscular activities and great angular velocities place the golfer at risk for incurring several injuries. Indeed this downswing period produces the greatest percentage of injuries in golfers today.[61,62] During these swing segments, increased stresses on the trunk and low back continue if improper spinal angles remain.

In a study conducted by Glazebrook et al,[68] EMG analysis of the forearm muscles revealed that the golfers with symptoms of medial epicondylitis displayed a greater activity of the wrist flexor muscles in the trailing arm during acceleration. These authors described the increased activity as an overloading force that may predispose the golfer to develop tendinopathy of the medial forearm musculotendinous structures.

Another potential source of injury occurs as the clubhead approaches ball contact. At this point, the speed and energy generated from the body are transferred through the wrist and hand into the clubhead.[70] The small bones of the wrist and hand are prone to injury if contact is made with the turf or other semiyielding surfaces.

Rotational forces continue in the trunk during the follow-through phases of the golf swing. Knowing that the follow-through position should be a mirror image of the downswing, golfers often overcompensate trunk movements to mimic that posture. As a result, physical loads on the spine are increased. As the swing continues to late follow-through, symptoms of pain may be experienced in the lead shoulder as it is placed in maximal amounts of external rotation.[69] As previously described, knee injuries and ankle sprains can result in the follow-through phases. Follow-through accounts for up to 30% of swing-related injuries to professional golfers; therefore, it should not be overlooked when evaluating the golf swing.

Golfers should be aware of the potential risks involved in the game of golf. The golf swing is an unnatural movement and inherently places significant stresses on the human body. The role of proper body mechanics, adequate strength and flexibility, and sufficient trunk stabilization simply cannot be overemphasized.

## Modifications to the Golf Swing

Many golfers with orthopedic problems tinker with their swings to reduce strain on vulnerable parts. Here we provide viable swing alterations that allow the golfer to participate in the game of golf in a more safe and effective manner. Common injuries and pain patterns will be discussed with suggestions on possible adjustments to the swing.

One of the most common strategies to decrease stresses on the spine is to shorten the swing, to reduce twisting of the trunk and spine. A study by Bulbulian et al[71] suggests that shortening the backswing may have a beneficial impact on the trunk, and by implication, reduce the potential for back problems. They found that the shortened backswing did reduce trunk muscle activation, without reducing clubhead velocity or ball-contact accuracy. However, the golfer may attempt to compensate for the shortened backswing through excessive arm movement or overactivation. This may be detrimental to the

shoulders. The rehab professional should monitor this closely and stress that the backswing is ultimately being shortened for the overall benefit of the golfer.

As noted earlier, the golfer's spine flexion angle at setup must be evaluated and corrected as needed. The most common mistake at setup is the use of forward flexion at the spine, instead of the proper hip-hinge. When a proper hip-hinge is used, the golfer flexes through the hip and allows for maintenance of a neutral spine.

The length of the golf club affects the level of stress on the spine during the golf swing. Research has provided evidence that different clubs produce different trunk motion characteristics.[70] When comparing the spine angles that resulted from the golf swing using a 7 iron versus a driver, increased spinal flexion and side bending occurred with the shorter 7 iron. Therefore, club length modifications may aid in the prevention or control of low back pain as well as injury to other segments in the kinetic chain.

## Rehabilitation, Conditioning, and Training Tips for Golfers

The primary goals for advancing a rehabilitation program for the golfer are injury prevention and performance enhancement. A proper conditioning and training routine will not only help to prevent further injuries, but it will enhance performance and prolong the golfer's playing career. Indeed, investigations by Fletcher and Hartwell[72] and Thompson and Osness[73] both revealed that appropriate strengthening and conditioning routines improve clubhead speed and driving distance. Flexibility also improved without an increase in spinal torque in recreational golfers following an 8-week conditioning program.

The components of a successful conditioning and training program include proper warm-up, flexibility, strength, power, skill training, and cardiovascular conditioning. If the golfer fails to train each component, optimal performance may not be achieved and injuries may occur.

To both prevent injury and improve performance, there are several basic conditioning and training principles that should followed when developing a program for the golfer.[74]

1. *The golfer should condition the entire body, not just the upper body.* Energy and power come from the legs, trunk, and hips during the golf swing.
2. *The exercise program should train each muscle as it functions during the golf swing.* For example, the large muscles of the upper extremities act as accelerators, and the rotator cuff and scapular muscles work primarily to stabilize and decelerate during the golf swing.
3. *The arms should be trained to act in concert with the legs/hips/trunk muscles.* The rotational components of legs/hips/trunk muscles act to enhance clubhead speed through the upper extremities during the golf swing.
4. *Core stability must be enhanced to provide for optimal swing patterns.* Correct postural alignment and a stable base of support provided by the hips, abdominal muscles, spinal stabilizers, and scapular muscles allow the proper swing path to occur.
5. *The golfer must train for bilateral strength.* The left and right sides of the body provide vital contributions and should not be neglected.
6. *Muscular strength is emphasized before dynamic strength and power.* A base level of strength is needed before more dynamic and powerful activities can be initiated.
7. *Muscular strength and flexibility are dependent upon each other for success.* Without the other, strength or flexibility cannot be utilized in an optimal manner.
8. *Conditioning and training should be performed year-round and should be periodized.* The golfer should allow for a year-round commitment to training and should vary training volumes and intensities in a systematic manner throughout the year.

Although expensive gym machines, intricate and detailed routines, and other gimmicks are available, a conditioning and training program does not always need to be elaborate. Home-based programs incorporating bodyweight, light dumbbells, weighted clubs, or elastic tubing resistance can be utilized.

## Proper Warm-up for Golfers

Preparing the body before play benefits performance and decreases the risk of injury.

However, when investigating the warm-up practices of golfers, it was found that only 54.3% performed some form of warm-up activity.[75] Air-swings on the tee were the most commonly observed warm-up exercise. This is hardly a proper routine. Fradkin et al[76] demonstrated that a proper warm-up routine actually increased clubhead speed when performed. Gosheger et al[77] found that a warm-up routine of at least 10 minutes in duration had a positive effect on the reduction of golfing injuries.

An appropriate warm-up for golfers should include a period of exercise to increase body temperature, followed by active stretching of the "golf muscles" (hands, wrists, forearms, shoulders, lower back, chest, trunk, hamstrings, and groin). The following outline will appropriately prepare the golfer to play and hopefully allow for decreased injury rates and improved performance.

1. *General warm-up.* The first goal of a warm-up routine should be to raise the body's core temperature. As body temperature increases, so does the ability to produce force.
2. *Mobility drills.* Mobility training increases the blood flow to the joints, "lubricates" them, and keeps their surfaces smooth and healthy.
3. *Dynamic flexibility.* Once the core temperature has increased and the joints are lubricated, dynamic stretches should be performed. It is important to start each dynamic stretch with a limited range of motion and then gradually increase the range. If you force a muscle into a new range by building up too much momentum, your dynamic stretching can backfire. Forcing a muscle into an extreme range too quickly will trigger the stretch reflex and your muscles will contract instead of relax.
4. *Skill progression.* Before moving on to the first tee, a series of golf swings with a progressive increase in range of motion and vigor should be performed.

## Interval Golf Program

To safely and effectively allow for return to unrestricted participation in golfing, the golfer must allow for a gradual application of forces to the involved healing structures. The interval golf program (**Table 9–7**) is simply an outline

**Table 9–7**   Interval Golf Program

|  | Day 1 | Day 2 | Day 3 |
|---|---|---|---|
| Week 1 | 10 putts<br>10 chips<br>Rest<br>15 chips | 15 putts<br>15 chips<br>Rest<br>25 chips | 20 putts<br>20 chips<br>Rest<br>20 putts<br>20 chips<br>Rest<br>10 chips<br>10 short irons |
| Week 2 | 20 chips<br>10 short irons<br>Rest<br>10 short irons | 20 chips<br>15 short irons<br>Rest<br>10 short irons<br>15 chips | 15 short irons<br>10 med irons<br>Rest<br>20 short irons<br>15 chips |
| Week 3 | 15 short irons<br>10 med irons<br>Rest<br>5 long irons<br>15 short Irons<br>Rest<br>20 chips | 15 short irons<br>10 med irons<br>10 long irons<br>Rest<br>10 short irons<br>10 med irons<br>5 long irons<br>5 woods | 15 short irons<br>10 med irons<br>10 long irons<br>Rest<br>10 short irons<br>10 med irons<br>10 long irons<br>10 woods |
| Week 4 | 15 short irons<br>10 med irons<br>10 long irons<br>10 drives<br>Rest<br>Repeat above | Play 9 holes | Play 9 holes |
| Week 5 | Play 9 holes | Play 9 holes | Play 18 holes |

**Key to golf program:**
Chips – pitching wedge
Short irons – W, 9, 8
Medium irons – 7, 6, 5
Long irons – 4, 3, 2
Woods – 3, 5
Drives – driver

**Guidelines:**
1. Always pay attention to the mechanics of your golf swing.
2. Allow one day of rest between sessions.
3. Perform a thorough and complete body warm-up and active stretching routine before training.
4. You must perform the program as outlined for each day without complications before advancing to the next step.
5. Although minor discomfort is expected intermittently, avoid swinging the golf club if it causes pain.

*If pain and or swelling persist, discontinue the program until examined by a medical professional. Resume the program at the step preceding the offending step.*

Adapted from Reinold MM, Wilk KE, Reed J, et al. Interval sports programs: guidelines for baseball, tennis, and golf. J Orthop Sports Phys Ther 2002;32:298, Table 7. Adapted by permission.

that provides for this gradual progression of forces and helps to prevent the eager golfer from doing "too much too soon."

Before initiating the interval golf program, the golfing athlete must satisfy several criteria. The individual should possess satisfactory ROM and mobility, minimal pain and tenderness, proper dynamic stabilization, and sufficient strength for the golf swing.[78] The table provided outlines a 5-week golfing progression. Stresses are steadily increased by progressing the golf clubs used—from short irons to medium irons to long irons. Eventually, the long irons progress to fairway woods and drivers.

## ◆ Summary

The interval sport return programs and guidelines reviewed in this chapter are meant to provide guidance to clinicians when returning patients to these sports following shoulder injury. In each sport section, we also outlined key challenges with respect to the GH and ST joints inherent in the sport-specific patterning and functions. This information provides key insights into the often-overlooked final phase of the rehabilitation process and encourages the clinician to integrate biomechanical information and sport science research with the patient's clinical presentation to facilitate this important final process.

## References

1. Hamner DL, Pink MM, Jobe FW. A modification of the relocation test: arthroscopic findings associated with a positive test. J Shoulder Elbow Surg 2000;9:263–267
2. Ellenbecker TS. Clinical Examination of the Shoulder. Philadelphia, PA: Elsevier Saunders; 2004
3. Ellenbecker TS, Davies GJ. The application of isokinetics in testing and rehabilitation of the shoulder complex. J Athletic Training 2000;35:338–350
4. Ellenbecker T, Roetert EP. Age specific isokinetic glenohumeral internal and external rotation strength in elite junior tennis players. J Sci Med Sport 2003; 6:63–70
5. Wilk KE, Andrews JR, Arrigo CA, Keirns MA, Erber DJ. The strength characteristics of the internal and external rotator muscles in professional baseball pitchers. Am J Sports Med 1993;21:61–69
6. Kibler WB. The role of the scapula in athletic shoulder function. Am J Sports Med 1998;26:325–337
7. Hanavan EP Jr. A mathematical model of the human body. AMRL-TR-64-102. AMRL TR 1964;18:64–102
8. Davies GJ. A Compendium of Isokinetics in Clinical Usage and Rehabilitation Techniques. 4th ed. Onalaska, WI: S & S Publishing; 1992
9. Putnam CA. Sequential motions of the body segments in striking and throwing skills: descriptions and explanations. J Biomech 1993;26(Suppl 1):125–136
10. Bunn J. Scientific Principles of Coaching. Englewood Cliffs, NJ: Prentice Hall; 1972
11. Kreighbaum E, Barthels KM. Biomechanics: A Qualitative Approach for Studying Human Movement. Minneapolis, MN: Burgess; 1985
12. Plagenhoef S. Patterns of Human Movement. Englewood Cliffs, NJ: Prentice Hall; 1971
13. Marshall RN, Elliott BC. Long-axis rotation: the missing link in proximal to distal sequencing. J Sports Sci 2000;18:247–254
14. Vaughan RE. An algorithm for determining arm action during overarm baseball pitches. In: Winter DA, Norman RW, Wells RP, Patla AE, eds. Biomechanics. Champaign, IL: Human Kinetics Publishers; 1985: 510–515
15. Joris HJJ, Edwards van Muyen AJ, Van Ingen Shenau GJ, Kemper HCG. Force, velocity and energy flow during the overarm throw in female handball players. J Biomech 1985;18:409–414
16. Ishii K, Suzuki M, Saito Y, Muira K, Fukinaga H. Contribution factors to increase velocity of a distal end in human body: ball throwing. In: Adrian M, Deutch H, eds. Biomechanics: The 1984 Olympic Scientific Congress Proceedings. Eugene, OR: Microform Publications; 1986:87–93
17. Elliott B, Marsh T, Blanksby B. A three dimensional cinematographic analysis of the tennis serve. Int J Sport Biomechanics 1986;2:260–271
18. VanGheluwe B, Hebbelinck M. The kinematics of the service movement in tennis: a three dimensional cinematographical approach. In Winter DA, Norman RW, Wells RP, Patla AE, eds. Biomechanics. Champaign, IL: Human Kinetics;1985:521–526
19. Feltner ME, Depena J. Dynamics of the shoulder and elbow joints of the throwing arm during a baseball pitch. Int J Sport Biomechanics 1986;2:235–259
20. Springings E, Marshall R, Elliott B, Jennings L. A three-dimensional kinematic method for determining the effectiveness of arm segment rotations in producing racquet head speed. J Biomech 1994;27:245–254
21. Groppel JL. High Tech Tennis. 2nd ed. Champaign, IL: Human Kinetics Publishers; 1992
22. Kibler WB. Clinical biomechanics of the elbow in tennis: Implications for evaluation and diagnosis. Med Sci Sports Exerc 1994;26:1203–1206
23. Ryu KN, McCormick J, Jobe FW, et al. An electromyographic analysis of shoulder function in tennis players. Am J Sports Med 1988;16:481–485
24. Dillman CJ, Fleisig GS, Werner SL, Andrews JR: Biomechanics of the shoulder in sports: throwing activities. Postgraduate studies in sports physical therapy. Berryville, VA: Forum Medicum, Inc; 1991:1–9
25. Shapiro R, Stine RL. Shoulder rotation velocities. Technical report submitted to the Lexington Clinic, Lexington, KY; 1992
26. Burkhart SS, Morgan CD, Kibler WB. The disabled throwing shoulder: spectrum of pathology, I: Pathoanatomy and biomechanics. Arthroscopy 2003; 19:404–420
27. Ellenbecker TS. Rehabilitation of shoulder and elbow injuries in tennis players. Clin Sports Med 1995;14: 87–110

28. Ellenbecker TS, Roetert EP, Piorkowski PA, Schulz DA. Glenohumeral joint internal and external rotation range of motion in elite junior tennis players. J Orthop Sports Phys Ther 1996;24:336–341

29. Kibler WB, Chandler TJ, Livingston BP, Roetert EP. Shoulder range of motion in elite tennis players. Am J Sports Med 1996;24:279–285

30. Roetert EP, Groppel J. World Class Tennis Technique. Champaign IL: Human Kinetics Publishers; 2001

31. Segal DK. Tenis Sistema Biodinamico. Buenos Aires, Argentina: Tenis Club Argentino; 2002

32. Giangarra CE, Conroy B, Jobe FW, et al. Electromyographic and cinematographic analysis of elbow function in tennis players using single- and double-handed backhand strokes. Am J Sports Med 1993; 21:394–399

33. Roetert EP, Brody H, Dillman CJ, Groppel JL, Schultheis JM. The Biomechanics of Tennis Elbow. Clin Sports Med 1995;14:47–58

34. Fleisig GS, Andrews JR, Dillman CJ, Escamilla RF. Kinetics of baseball pitching with implications about injury mechanisms. Am J Sports Med 1995;23: 233–239

35. Glousman R, Jobe FW, Tibone JE, et al. Dynamic electromyographic analysis of the throwing shoulder with glenohumeral joint instability. J Bone Joint Surg Am 1988;70-A:220–226

36. Fleisig GS, Dillman CJ, Andrews JR. Proper mechanics for baseball pitching. Clin Sports Med 1989;1:1 51–170

37. Atwater AE. Biomechanics of overarm throwing movements and of throwing injuries. Exerc Sport Sci Rev 1979;7:43–85

38. Fleisig GS, Escamilla RF, Barrentine SW, Zheng N, Andrews JR. Kinematic and kinetic comparison of baseball pitching from a mound and throwing from flat ground. Paper presented at: The Twentieth Annual Meeting of the American Society of Biomechanics, October 17–19, 1996; Atlanta, GA

39. Fleisig GS, Zheng N, Barrentine SW, Escamilla RF, Andrews JR, Lemak LJ. Kinematic and kinetic comparison of full-effort and partial-effort baseball pitching. Paper presented at: The Twentieth Annual Meeting of the American Society of Biomechanics, October 17–19, 1996; Atlanta, GA

40. Wilk KE, Arrigo CA, Andrews JR. The abductor and adductor strength characteristics of professional baseball pitchers. Am J Sports Med 1995;23:307–311

41. Wilk KE, Arrigo CA. Current concepts in the rehabilitation of the athlete shoulder. J Orthop Sports Phys Ther 1993;18:365–378

42. Wilk KE, Reinold MM, Andrews JR. Postoperative treatment principles in the throwing athlete. Sports Med Arthrosc Rev 2001;9:69–95

43. Wilk KE, Andrews JR, Arrigo CA, et al. Preventive and rehabilitative exercises for the shoulder and elbow. 6th ed. Birmingham, AL: American Sports Medicine Institute; 2001

44. Johnson JE, Sim FH, Scott SG. Musculoskeletal injuries in competitive swimmers. Mayo Clin Proc 1987;62: 289–304

45. Kennedy JC, Craig AB, Schneider RC. Swimming. In: Schneider RC, Kennedy JC, Plant ML, eds. Sports Injuries: Mechanisms, Prevention and Treatment. Baltimore, MD: Williams & Wilkins; 1985

46. Kennedy JC, Hawkins R, Krissoff WB. Orthopaedic manifestations of swimming. Am J Sports Med 1978;6:309–322

47. McMaster WC, Troup J. A survey of interfering shoulder pain in United States competitive swimmers. Am J Sports Med 1993;21:67–70

48. Greipp JF. Swimmer's shoulder: the influence of flexibility and weight training. Phys Sportsmed 1985; 13:92–105

49. Kammer S, Young CC, Niedfeldt MW. Swimming Injuries and Illnesses. Phys Sportsmed 1999;27:51–60

50. Colwin CM. Swimming Into the 21st Century. Champaign, IL: Human Kinetics Publishers; 1992

51. Costill DL, Maglischo EW, Richardson AB. Handbook of Sports Medicine and Science: Swimming. Oxford: Blackwell Scientific Publications; 1992

52. Councilman JG. The Science of Swimming. Englewood Cliffs, NJ: Prentice Hall; 1968

53. Maglischo EW. Swimming Faster. Palo Alto, CA: Mayfield; 1982

54. Falkel JE, Murphy TC. Shoulder injuries. In: Malone T, ed. Sports Injury Management Series. Baltimore, MD: Williams & Wilkins; 1988

55. Murphy TC. Shoulder injuries in swimming. In: Andrews JR, Wilk KE, eds. The Athlete's Shoulder. New York, NY: Churchill Livingstone; 1994

56. Murphy TC, Riester JN. Managing the young swimmer: a practical approach to prevention and treatment. The Student Athlete 1988;1:4–8

57. Penny JN, Smith C. The prevention and treatment of swimmer's shoulder. Can J Appl Sport Sci 1980;5: 195–202

58. Russ DW. A case report: in-season management of shoulder pain in a collegiate swimmer–A team approach. (abstract) J Orthop Sports Phys Ther 1997; 25:86

59. Miburm PD. Summation of segmental velocities in the golf swing. Med Sci Sports Exerc 1982;32:60–64

60. Mallarc C. Golf's contribution to low back pain. Sports Med Update 1997;11:20–25

61. McCarroll JR, Gioe TJ. Professional golfers and the price they pay. Phys Sportsmed 1982;10:64–70

62. Duda M. Golf injuries: They really do happen. Phys Sportsmed 1987;15:190–196

63. Gosheger G, Liem D, Ludwig K, Greshake O, Winkelmann W. Injuries and overuse syndromes in golf. Am J Sports Med 2003;31:438–443

64. Pink M, Perry J, Jobe FW. Electromyographic analysis of the trunk in golfers. Am J Sports Med 1993;21: 385–388

65. Pink M, Jobe FW, Perry J. Electromyographic analysis of the shoulder during a golf swing. Am J Sports Med 1990;18:137–140

66. Kao JT, Pink M, Jobe FW. Electromyographic analysis of the scapular muscles during a golf swing. Am J Sports Med 1995;23:19–23

67. Jobe FW, Moynes DR, Antonelli DJ. Rotator cuff function during a golf swing. Am J Sports Med 1986; 14:388–392

68. Glazebrook MA, Curwin S, Islam MN, et al. Medial epicondylitis: an electromyographic analysis and an investigation of intervention strategies. Am J Sports Med 1994;22:674–679

69. Mallon WJ. Golf. In: Hawkins RJ, Misamore GW, eds. Shoulder Injuries in the Athlete. New York, NY: Churchill Livingstone; 1996 pp. 427–433

70. Geisler P. Kinesiology of the full golf swing: implications for intervention and rehabilitation. Sports Med Update 1997;11:9–19

71. Bulbulian R, Ball KA, Seaman DR. The short golf back-swing: effects on performance and spinal health implications. J Manipulative Physiol Ther 2001;24:569–575

72. Fletcher IM, Hartwell M. Effect of an 8-week combined weights and plyometrics training program on golf drive performance. J Strength Cond Res 2004;18:59–62

73. Thompson CJ, Osness WH. Effects of an 8-week multimodal exercise program on strength, flexibility, and golf performance in 55- to 79-year-old men. J Aging Phys Act 2004;12:144–156

74. Wilk KE. Conditioning and training techniques. In: Hawkins RJ, Misamore GW, eds. Shoulder Injuries in the Athlete. New York, NY: Churchill Livingstone; 1996 pp. 339–363

75. Fradkin AJ, Sherman CA, Finch CF. Improving golf performance with a warm up conditioning programme. Br J Sports Med 2004;38:762–765

76. Fradkin AJ, Finch CF, Sherman CA. Warm-up attitudes and behaviours of amateur golfers. J Sci Med Sport 2003;6:210–215

77. Gosheger G, Liem D, Ludwig K, Greshake O, Winkelmann W. Injuries and overuse syndromes in golf. Am J Sports Med 2003;31:438–443

78. Reinold MM, Wilk KE, Reed J, Crenshaw K, Andrews JR. Interval sport programs: guidelines for baseball, tennis, and golf. J Orthop Sports Phys Ther 2002;32:293–298

# Index

Page numbers followed by *f* or *t* indicate figures and tables, respectively.

Grip type, for weightlifting, 110–113, 111*f*–113*f*
Groundstrokes, in tennis, 142–144

## H

Hand spacing, for weightlifting, 110, 111*f*, 112–116
Hawkins impingement test, 6
Heat therapy, for adhesive capsulitis, 67–68
High-five position, in weightlifting, 108, 109*f*
Hill-Sachs lesions, 42
Hip flexibility, in golf swing, 159–160
Hip/trunk stability, in scapular dyskinesis, 100, 100*f*
Hockey players, brace effectiveness in, 131
Hooked acromion (type III), 4–5
Horizontal abduction, prone
    for acromioclavicular joint injury, 90, 90*f*
    for rotator cuff strengthening, 12–13, 12*f*
    in Thrower's Ten Program, 31*f*–32*f*
Horizontal adduction stretch, 28, 28*f*
Hyperangulation, in tennis players, 142

## I

Ice
    for acromioclavicular joint injury, 80–81
    for micro-instability, 29
Immobilization
    for acromioclavicular joint injury, 79–80, 79*f*
    in adduction and internal rotation, 42–45, 50
    analogy to ACL treatment, 43
    braces available for, 42–43, 43*f*
    for dislocation/instability, 42–45
    in external rotation, 44–45, 45*f*
    functional outcome of, 44–45
    past and present approaches in, 42–45
    recurrence rate after, 42–44
    standard of care in, 43
    taping or strapping for, 43
    UltraSling for, 45, 45*f*
    in younger *versus* older patients, 42
Impingement, 4–20
    acromial architecture in, 4–5
    anterior internal, 6
    blood flow in, improvement of, 6
    braces for, 136
    discharge considerations in, 18–19
    functional indexes or rating scales in, 19
    internal, 5–6, 25, 25*f*
    isokinetic exercises for, 15–16, 17*f*
    isometric exercises for, 6–7
    mobilization techniques for, 7–9, 11
    Neer's stages of, 4–5
    outcomes of nonoperative treatment in, 19–20
    outlet, 4

posterior, 5–6
posterior drawer test in, 8, 8*f*
primary (compressive disease), 4–5
range of motion in
    assessment of, 7–9, 8*f*
    improvement/strengthening of, 11–18
    total, concept of, 9–11
rehabilitation of, 6–19
    dynamometer use in, 16
    initial phase of, 6–11
    total arm strength phase of, 11–18
resistive exercise for, 11–20
scapular dyskinesis in, 98
scapular stabilization for, 6–7
    manual techniques of, 6–7, 7*f*
    rhythmic, 7, 7*f*
secondary, 5
stage 1 (edema and hemorrhage), 4
stage II (compressive disease), 4
stage III (bone spurs and tendon rupture), 4
strengthening exercises for, 11–18
    closed chain, 13–14, 14*f*, 18, 18*f*
    external oscillation, 13, 13*f*
    external rotation in standing (with towel roll), 13, 13*f*
    external rotation with retraction, 13, 14*f*
    90/90 external rotation, 12*f*, 13
    plus position, 13–14, 14*f*–15*f*
    plyometric, 16–18, 17*f*–18*f*
    pointer position, 13, 15*f*
    primary goals of, 12
    progression of, 12*f*
    prone extension, 12, 12*f*
    prone horizontal abduction, 12–13, 12*f*
    side-lying external rotation, 12, 12*f*
stretching for
    home programs of, 11, 11*f*
    passive, 10–11, 10*f*
submaximal exercise for, 6–7
    in swimmers, 6, 151–152
taping in, 128–130, 129*t*
types of, 4–6
undersurface, 5–6, 25, 25*f*
Infraspinatus muscle, in golf swing, 156–159
Instability, 40–60
    ACL analogy of, 43, 56
    AMBRI and, 40–42
    anterior drawer test for, 26, 27*f*, 47*f*
    anterior fulcrum test for, 26–27, 27*f*
    Bankart lesions with, 42
    braces for, 42–43, 43*f*, 130–131, 135*f*
    causes of, assessment of, 45–50
    circle concept and, 45
    classification of, 41–42
        American Shoulder and Elbow Society's, 46, 47*t*